WHO TAUGHT YOU THAT?

Answers to
101 Important Questions
About SEX

Dr. Leah M. Schwartz

WHO TAUGHT YOU THAT?

Answers to 101 Important Questions About SEX

Copyright ©2002
by Leah M. Schwartz, Ph.D.

ISBN: 0-942540-75-1
Library of Congress PCN: 2002095017

Published by Breakthru Publishing
P.O. Box 2866, Houston, TX 77252

Printed in Canada

Acknowledgments

First and foremost, I would like to thank Dr. W. Victor Baranco. Without his phenomenal wisdom and insight into human sexuality, this book would not have been possible. Though Dr. Baranco is no longer with us, his words continue to provide inspiration and guidance. And for their generosity and graciousness, I wish to also thank Drs. Cynthia Baranco and Suzanne Baranco, who were active partners in his life-long research.

I especially want to thank:

My Mother Her words, "a heart feels a heart," touch my life everyday and inspire me to go on. I am so grateful that she is my Mom. There are no words to express the power of a Mother's Love.

Janet O'Neal Thank you for being in my life and for believing in me; for your unconditional love, support, wisdom and for all your encouragement. You have always been there for me when I needed you. I am so honored to call you my best friend and sister. You are the wind beneath my wings.

Melva Hemphill I am blessed to have you in my life, thank you for letting me know I could call you anytime, day or night. Your commitment to people's relationships and making this a better place to live inspires me everyday. Thank you for your unconditional love and support.

Luz Maya My gratitude goes out to you, my cherished friend for being there for me day in and day out, being a constant reminder of how blessed we are to do God's work and that God is with us always.

Jack Mayer For your total commitment and dedication and support in empowering this book to be the best it could be, for your extraordinary eye in designing, layout, type and for final editing.

John Martin Thank you for helping me organize my thoughts, and for being a good ear for what my vision for this book is.

Thanks to my dear and true friend, *Walter Maksym*, who has been a friend, attorney and advisor to Breakthru Publishing, the late Dr. Victor Baronco and More University, and my late husband; for assisting me with this book and for his unconditional love, encouragement and support during my most difficult time.

Statement of Purpose

My purpose in writing this book was simple: to educate readers in the relationship philosophy and skills necessary for a more pleasurable, fulfilling and fun sex life. For many, the information divulged in these pages may fly in the face of beliefs accepted without question for almost as long as people have been discussing the subject of sex. In fact, that is one purpose of this work: to question superstitious beliefs about sex and relationships that have long been held sacred in our society, but have often done more harm than good. The challenge I faced was to contest these beliefs while maintaining a spirit of respect for those who hold them. I trust that this book meets that challenge.

If this work helps my readers reconsider even one piece of detrimental "conventional wisdom" about sex, it will be far more than a victory; it will be a major step toward their own sexual fulfillment. That is the ultimate purpose of all my work.

Dedication

Who Taught You That? is dedicated in loving memory to my late husband, Dr. Bob Schwartz, whose unshakable faith in the potentialities of monogamous relationships continues to support and fortify me as I go forward without him.

The perfected spiritual union between two people is a wondrous and rare thing, and no better expression of that union exists than in the act of lovemaking. This book carries on the work begun in our previous book, The One Hour Orgasm, addressing important questions asked by couples as they explore, or in some cases, work through, the problems involved in achieving true intimacy. In attempting to answer these questions for the benefit of readers everywhere, I know that Dr. Bob was always there with me, guiding whenever I faltered, hanging back when I soared, fulfilling the role of companion and husband, just as he always had done.

 Thank you, Dr. Bob—I love you.

Nothing can replace the loss of a life partner, but in continuing the excellent work that my husband and I began together, I hope to extend that legacy, and, in time, come to see intimacy in ways I now only imagine—necessarily changed, as they must be, and as I must learn to accept.

This book is a starting point only…but it is my fondest hope that it is the beginning of an exciting and fulfilling journey for you and your partner.

Dr. Leah M. Schwartz

Houston, Texas
December 2002

I Think There's Something Wrong With Me

1 *I am thirty-one years old and have never climaxed during intercourse. I have come what I thought was very close. What can I/we do to change this? I also notice that the more I have sex, the easier it is for me to become aroused. But during extended absences, my body seems to go to sleep. As much as I would like to get in the mood, my body awakens too slowly.*

The goal of relating with your partner sensually is to experience pleasure. The idea that intercourse is the right way for men and women to achieve gratification has resulted in people becoming goal-oriented rather than pleasure-oriented in their relationships. Any way that feels good to you is right. The way to get aroused is to take pleasure in whatever you're doing. Judging and measuring yourself is not a turn-on.

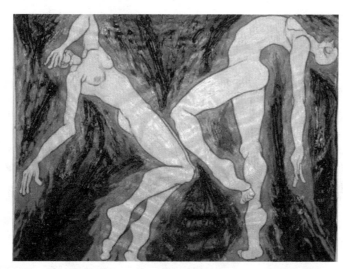

Who Taught You *That*?

2 *I am in my twenties, and rarely orgasm during sex. However, I always climax when I pleasure myself. Is there something wrong with my state of mind during sex, or is it that I don't know myself as well as I thought I did?*

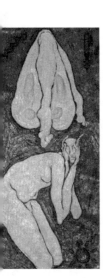

There is nothing wrong with you. Actually, it is just the opposite. It is wonderful that you know how you like to be touched and know where, when, and how to do so. The good news is that you know you can have orgasms, and that you do have them. The fact that you do not have them during intercourse is common for most women because in most cases, your most sensitive part is not getting touched.

When you start to have intercourse, you may not immediately feel the feelings you normally experience when you pleasure yourself, causing you to compare the experience you're having with experiences you've had in the past, which can then take you "out of" the experience. Another thing that could be happening is that you may not be engorged when you start intercourse, which prevents your most sensitive part (your clitoris) from being properly stimulated. What I suggest is that you show your lover how to touch you the way that you like, and then try some new positions until you find a position you like better.

You know yourself well enough. It is your lovers who do not know you as well as they should. Men rarely hear complaints from women, let alone good instruction. If you don't teach your lovers the proper way to stimulate you, they will go on to the next sexual experience being as inept as before. Why not teach them the right way to do it? Even if this relationship eventually breaks up, you'll be doing the next girl a favor.

Dr. Leah M. Schwartz

3 *My boyfriend and I have been together for five years, and the only way he's ever been able to make me reach climax is to gently suck my breasts. Is there something wrong with me? Until he sucks my breasts, I can go for hours without ever reaching climax.*

No; there is nothing wrong with you. Your whole nervous system is connected, and one of the connections where you are most sensitive is the connection between your breast area and clitoris. Your lover, however, can learn when and how to touch you without touching your breasts and then, as you start to feel those other good feelings, he can begin to stimulate your breasts to intensify those feelings. There are many ways to reach a climax. Having discovered one way, you can now explore what other ways are available to you. Theoretically, it is possible to achieve climax anywhere on your body.

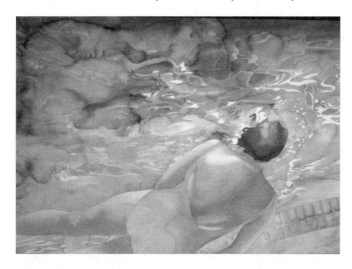

Who Taught You *That*?

4 *Since I had a hysterectomy, I can't seem to get enough sex. I could have sex twenty-four hours a day, but I have no takers. What can I do?*

What you can do is investigate your own genitalia. Rub yourself inside your vaginal walls and around your vulva. Feel how varied your responses are, and discover that your clitoris is the most sensitive part of your genitalia. Pull back the hood of your clitoris and with a lubricated finger (Petroleum-based Vaseline® is best for this, but should only be used for surface stimulation since it is not absorbed by the skin and doesn't evaporate) rub the head of your clitoris using varying pressure on different spots until you discover what area, pressure and speed gives you the most pleasure. Continue rubbing and, if the pleasurable sensation begins to fade, adjust the pressure and velocity until it feels as good as you can achieve.

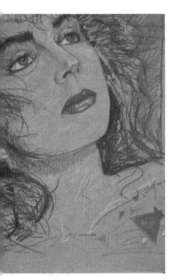

Practice this on a regular basis until you know what pleasures you the most. Teach your lover how you please yourself, and when your lover has become competent, relax and enjoy it. You will find yourself to be quite satiable.

Many women who rely solely on intercourse for gratification believe themselves to be insatiable. That's because intercourse is not an efficient way to achieve satisfaction. The freedom from fear of pregnancy that follows a hysterectomy or menopause often permits a woman to enjoy intercourse more than ever, but clitoral stimulation is still the best way to achieve satisfaction.

Dr. Leah M. Schwartz

5 *I have been dating my boyfriend for nine months now. When we have sex, I never achieve orgasm. I've never told him this. I have tried different things with him such as manipulating the positions we use, or having him perform oral sex, but nothing seems to work. He, on the other hand, has orgasms every single time. I can honestly say that I've never had an orgasm through vaginal intercourse. I have, however, had an orgasm from oral sex or masturbation. We are attracted to each other, and he can "turn me on." I desperately want to have an orgasm with him, but I've run out of ideas. He is older than me by eight years. Please help!*

Your comments are very common among women. The reason why he has an orgasm every time you have intercourse is because his most sensitive part is getting stimulated by rubbing inside you whereas in most cases, your most sensitive part (your clitoris) is not getting enough contact with the motion of his penis. It is possible for a woman to reach orgasm during intercourse if she's engorged enough and if you adjust your position so that his incursive motion strokes your clitoris. It will take some practice and cooperation to achieve this. Many women find that the woman-on-top position is best for achieving this because the woman knows when her clitoris is being stimulated. Intercourse is certainly not the best way for a woman, or a man, to reach orgasm, although in our society it is considered to be the major sexual act. Other activities are referred to as foreplay.

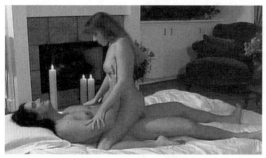

The best way for anyone to reach orgasm is to be relieved of the responsibility of producing sensation so that all of his or her attention is available for receiving and appreciating. Because you achieve orgasm from oral and manual sex, there is nothing wrong with enjoying intercourse for whatever pleasures it produces and achieving orgasm some other way. Your lover would obviously love to please you, and it's worth the investment to communicate with him about these matters.

6 *I am dating a guy who hasn't been with too many women, actually I am only his second and he's 27. He's been alone for so many years that he can only orgasm by touching himself—not from being with a woman. It's kind of frustrating, but there is just no way around it. I've done some research on the web and, short of sending him to a doctor, nothing they've suggested has seemed to do the trick. Do you know of any way to fix this problem, or what else we could try?*

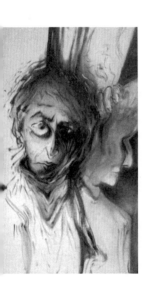

This is not really a problem, so it doesn't need to be fixed. Although many people feel if they don't have an orgasm, they have somehow failed. Orgasm is highly overrated. For most men it consists of six to nine contractions (spasms in the muscles around the base of the penis and the anus), spaced about a second apart. This means the average orgasm for a man lasts about six seconds, which is no big deal. The fun of sensuality is the pleasure that a person perceives in being stroked or rubbed, particularly in those areas of the body that contain the highest concentration of nerve endings. This pleasure is most fully experienced when the person's total attention is on his or her sensations. If you're trying to produce orgasm, then a lot of your attention is on whether or not you're going to succeed, whether you're getting closer or further away, etc. All of these considerations take attention away from what you're feeling at the moment, so you're missing a lot of the fun that contributes to an orgasm.

It's not only a matter of how many times you stroke him, but how many and how much of every stroke he actually feels. Your best move is to forget about orgasm for a while, let him know it doesn't matter to you, that he should just relax and pay attention to how good whatever stimulation he's getting—manual, genital, oral, etc.—feels. When you've had enough of doing whatever fun things you feel like, if he still wants an orgasm, encourage him to get himself off and participate in his self-administered pleasure in whatever way you both find fun.

Dr. Leah M. Schwartz

7 *I have not slept with anyone in the past couple of months. Recently, I met this guy and we hit it off really well. Eventually, we will become sexually active. In the past, whenever I have sex with someone for the first time, I normally do not enjoy it. Is there anything that I can do to be satisfied the first time around?*

Most important, don't do anything you don't want to do, or do it longer than you want to do it. There are many reasons for not enjoying yourself the first time. Your lover could be unskilled, or you could be bringing your past experience into this experience, creating expectations as to how you think it should be. Thus, your option is either to hope, or to teach him what feels good to you—the way you like to be touched.

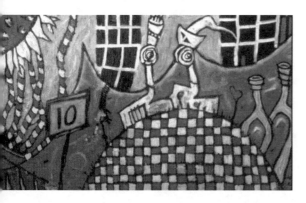

8 *I used to be able to reach orgasm very easily from oral sex or touching (never intercourse, unfortunately), but now it takes a lot more stimulation either from a vibrator or heavy pressure from my fingers. I wish it wasn't so difficult. I'm starting to wonder if I desensitized myself. Any suggestions/advice?*

When you were a sexual novice, you didn't know what to expect or how to achieve it, so when you finally stumbled across something that worked, it really swept you away, much as a first kiss could shake you to your shoes. Now that you have your own ideas as to what you should be able to achieve, you're always striving to attain these sensual goals. You've come across one way of getting there, constant heavy pressure. Unfortunately, the harder you try now, the more you interfere with and cancel out your progress.

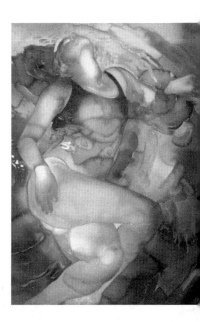

Not to worry—you still have the potential to respond to lighter, slower stroking. Set aside your need for quick, intense orgasms for a while. Occupy your mind with erotic thoughts, memories and images, and learn to enjoy the pleasures that you feel.

When you are rubbing on yourself and it starts to feel really good, instead of going harder and faster, slow down and lighten up, or even pause slightly before you start again. Take yourself "to the edge," then repeat the process until you build up such intensity that you can't stand it anymore. Only then take yourself over the edge. If it takes a long time, so much the better.

Dr. Leah M. Schwartz

9 *I am in a long-term relationship, and recently we have begun to have problems in the bedroom. I have multiple orgasms that ultimately cause me to be extremely wet—he, on the other hand, loses any sense of feeling/sensation during intercourse. Can you give me advice on how to resolve this?*

This problem has its origin in the idea that the best way for a man to reach orgasm is to pump a tight vagina. Widespread as this idea is, it isn't true. Manual and oral stimulation are capable of producing far more pleasure for a man than incursive motion in a lubricated hole.

If you want intercourse to be your principle sexual activity, there are a couple of things you can do. You can push down and out (as in defecation) during your orgasms. This will have the dual effect of spreading pleasurable sensations down your legs and up your torso and of tightening the channel of your vagina.

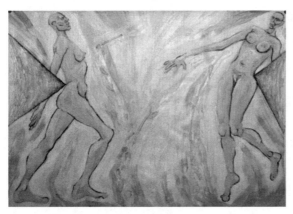

If you have ever sneezed during intercourse, you know that you can eject a penis from your vagina like toothpaste from a tube. That's an indication of the contracting power of the push out. Another thing you can do is have him put his legs on the outside with yours on the inside, while having intercourse in the missionary position. This will give you greater clitoral contact with the shaft of his penis and also tighten your vagina around his penis.

10

I would like to know how to stay wet during the time my lover and I have intercourse. I tend to dry out after about ten minutes.

A couple of things could be happening here. Either you are not enjoying yourself or you're spending too much time in your head wishing it were better. Be willing to just stop and use some lubricant. The harder you try to get lubricated, the harder it will be to achieve. If you are thinking about lubrication instead of your pleasure, you'll only make the situation worse. Many women experience dryness especially as they get older. There is no reason at all for you to suffer from dryness. Use as much water-soluble lubricant as necessary to feel comfortable.

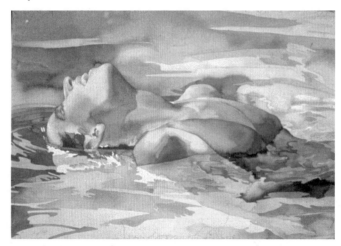

Dr. Leah M. Schwartz

11

I am a thirty-eight year old woman. Why, after eight years of marriage, am I dry?

If by "dry" you mean vaginally dry, it's probably menopause, or what is known as *peri-menopause*, even at 38. If you're experiencing vaginal dryness, you should see a doctor. Your vaginal dryness might not be accompanied by the cessation of menses, but your estrogen could be out of balance; or there might be some other cause for your consistent dryness such as anti-histamines.

In any case, it's important that you see a gynecologist. Until you do, use a water-soluble lubricant to relieve your discomfort and facilitate intercourse.

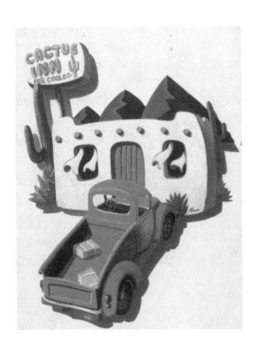

Who Taught You *That?*

12

Why is it painful when my husband makes love to me from a doggie-style position?

Some women report pain due to the head of the penis impacting the cervix (the neck of the womb that protrudes into the vaginal canal). In this case, if you push out and down as you do when emptying your bowels, it will have the effect of collapsing the vaginal walls around his penis and moving your cervix up and out of the line of his stroke. This will feel very good to him and should result in the head of his penis going into the pocket in front of your cervix called the *fornix*, which should increase your pleasure as well.

Communicate with your partner. Feel up inside yourself with your fingers so that you're aware of your anatomy and have him do the same so he understands it's not just an empty hole he's pumping into.

I also advise you to consult your gynecologist. If your doctor assures you that there is nothing wrong with you, you should be able to work it out so that you can experience lots of enjoyment doing it in this position.

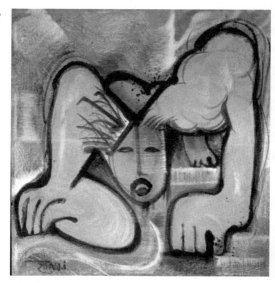

Dr. Leah M. Schwartz

13 *I am a woman, and I wondered why it takes so long to get lubricated?*

You are trying to drive the engine without warming it up. There is nothing wrong with the way that your body works—fill the time that you're waiting with activities that please you. If you're having sensual fun, why should you conclude that it's taking too long?

You don't have to be victimized by the time it takes you to lubricate. If you want to be lubricated before your body is ready, there are adequate lubricants on the market. If you could relax and use them, you might not need them. Performance anxiety isn't going to help.

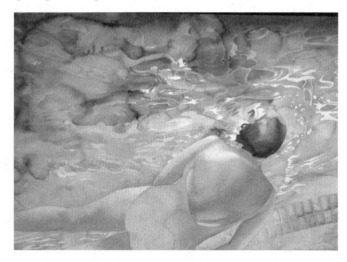

Who Taught You *That?*

14

It hurts when my husband and I have intercourse. Can you hurt yourself if you get sore from intercourse?

The answer to the second part of your question is—absolutely. It's a common myth in our society that harder and faster is the best way to pleasure or that it indicates how passionate or enthusiastic you are. In fact, it's the best way to get sore. Use an artificial lubricant, or lighten up.

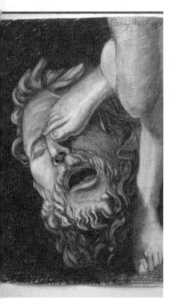

If any such pain persists, see a doctor. In regard to why your intercourse is painful I would definitely talk to your doctor about this. It could be due to a variety of physical or psychological reasons. You might not be sufficiently lubricated. In our society, many men consider their own engorgement sufficient to begin intercourse and ignore the woman's readiness. Take the time and attention to ensure that your own genitals are well-engorged and lubricated before you begin. Natural lubrication is at best unreliable in women and particularly with the approach of menopause. Do not hesitate to use water-soluble artificial lubricants. With menopause, the tissues lining the vagina thin out and can be more easily damaged.

The source of the pain could also be in your mind. Perhaps you are not looking forward to intercourse and, therefore, are not relaxed. Sensuality is about pleasuring one another's sensitive areas. If you are feeling pain, this is not sensuality.

Dr. Leah M. Schwartz

15 *How can I make myself comfortable enough to perform oral sex on my boyfriend? I want to bring him pleasure through oral sex as he does for me, but every time I think about it, I get scared or embarrassed. I feel as if I wouldn't know what to do.*

This is a dilemma for many women, and I understand how you feel. The best suggestion I can give you is simply to ask. In most cases, if you are honest about your lack of experience, it will actually be a turn on for him to go about teaching you.

Speed, direction, pressure and the lubrication supplied by your mouth will all become important factors in your technique. I would also tell you that it is okay to take breaks in between and start up again.

If you are put off by the idea of swallowing his ejaculate, simply leaving your lips slightly open so that the semen runs down his penis adds to the lubrication your saliva provides.

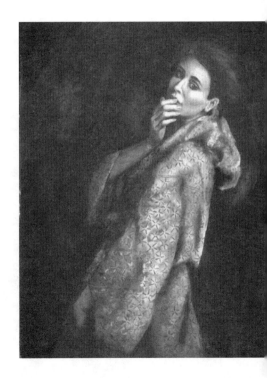

Who Taught You *That?*

16 *How come some men ask such stupid questions—questions such as: "How was it for you," "Did you have an orgasm?" and "Are you there yet?"*

These questions may seem stupid to you, but men in our society are conditioned to be performance-oriented and consequently, they pride themselves on how well they gratify their woman. They identify their own orgasm with their ejaculation, but unless the woman verbalizes or dramatizes her gratification, there is often no way for the man to know if he has successfully achieved his goal. Due to the widespread

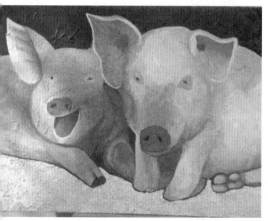

notion that intercourse is the best way for people to mutually gratify one another, some men pay little attention to the woman's clitoris. Previous lovers may also have faked gratification as a way of ending a sensual episode where there was fear of causing disappointment or starting an argument. The tone of your question suggests that you are not being fully satisfied. If you are lucky enough to be involved with a man who's interested in you, you could at least take advantage of the opportunity to teach him how to pleasure you more.

Dr. Leah M. Schwartz

17 *I can only reach climax when I cross my legs and squeeze/release. Why is this so, and how can I achieve this feeling when I am with my fiancé? Do I have a tilted uterus, or is there something wrong with me?*

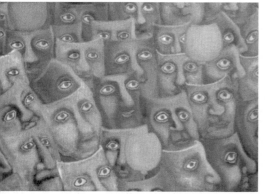

No, there is nothing wrong with you. The good news is that you know you can have orgasms. Now it is just a matter of teaching your lover how to touch you so that it feels the same as when you squeeze your own clitoris. The clitoris is that part of the human body that contains the highest concentration of nerve endings. As such, it is extremely sensitive and many women find that indirect stimulation such as that produced by flexing the thigh muscles is sufficient to produce an orgasm.

If you want your lover to provide you with a similar degree of pleasure, you must teach him the type and degree of pressure you find acceptable. The position of your uterus is irrelevant. Having a tilted uterus does not affect your orgasms. Your clitoris, which is the main source of your orgasm, is located on the outside of your sexual parts. Your uterus, of course, is on the inside. A tilted uterus, but not the activities you are describing, may affect different intercourse positions. Check with your gynecologist to see if you have a tilted uterus just so you know.

Who Taught You *That*?

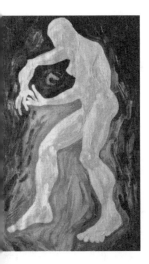

18

Why does my husband act as if he knows more about my body than I do?

He probably hasn't heard any complaints. Men are brought up in our society to believe that they should know something about everything. Traditionally, mothers would tell their daughters when asked what to expect on their wedding nights that their husbands would "know what to do." Your husband is afraid to look stupid. As with most men, he picked up most of what he knows about sex from his buddies at school, from pornography and from women who lied to him or told him that what he was doing brought pleasure to them because they did not want to deal with his ego or hurt feelings. In our culture, there is no systematic way for men to learn about women's bodies. Here is your opportunity to build on what he *does* know. Play a game called "show and tell" where you show him what you like while telling him verbally. Make it fun and easy and show him how he can win at pleasing you.

The first step is to acknowledge the actions or behaviors that already feel good. Second, make an easy request of him that will increase *your* pleasure such as "Would you go a little slower" or "Rub a little softer (or harder)" or "Come up a little higher (down a little lower)" or "Move your finger a little to the left (to the right)." Simple requests furnish him with the information he needs to be able to give you exactly what pleases you the most. The third step is to give him good feedback: "That is even better" or "That is wonderful" and "Oh, that is great, thank you!" Then go back to step one. To summarize:

Step 1. Acknowledge what is good.

Step 2. Make a small request he can fulfill.

Step 3. Acknowledge the improvement.

Repeat this communication cycle as many times as it continues to be productive and fun.

Dr. Leah M. Schwartz

19

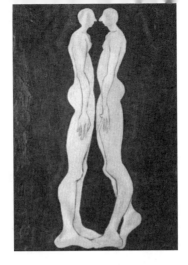

I have had few if any involuntary erections for some time. I think it dates back to my prostate surgery, which I think they screwed up. I've tried Viagra® and Muse® with no results, though I may have administered the latter improperly. All that's left to my knowledge is a penile implant, which I don't think I'll have, and a vacuum pump. I am seventy-four; my wife is seventy. I have very little difficulty reaching orgasm by masturbating, although sometimes I still have problems. Do you have any advice to offer me?

As long as you have an effective way to reach orgasm, the rest is unimportant. Involuntary erection is no indication of a man's capacity for sexual pleasure.

However, I'd venture to say that you could increase your enjoyment by being more open with your wife. Show her how you masturbate, and tell her the kind of fantasies you use to help you get there. If she wants to be further involved, try having your wife hold your penis with your hand around hers while she masturbates you.

If you would be more open with your wife, she might also be willing to be more open with her own techniques, and you could learn how to make the experience more satisfying for her as well. There is always room for improvement. You two could be having a lot more fun than you're already having—something that should keep you busy for the rest of your lives.

Who Taught You *That*?

20 *My girlfriend wants me to touch her clitoris directly, but she says when I do, it is too sensitive. What can I do?*

Take it as a compliment that she felt comfortable enough to make the request and that you in turn are willing to give her what she asked for. "Too sensitive" means very sensitive, which is good. Who would want a clitoris that is insensitive? What "too sensitive" means is "too sensitive for indiscriminate touching." It is your responsibility to discover her limits—the lightest and heaviest touches she can tolerate and enjoy. Schedule an investigative session with her in which your job will be to learn how to pleasure her the most. Agree ahead of time that the goal of the session will be for you to learn and for you both to have fun. Don't do it any longer than you both are enjoying it, and don't make orgasm your primary goal. Set the amount of time you intend to spend with an alarm clock or, alternatively, the duration of one CD.

As soon as the time is up, stop. Tell her how much fun you had and schedule a follow-up. Make the surroundings comfortable and attractive. Tell her all the things about her that please you—how pretty her hair is, how nice she smells and so on. Tell her what's next each step of the way, and let her know before completing each step that you're getting ready to stop.

Have her lie back and spread her legs. Apply a lubricant to your fingers that's been warmed up in your hands (I recommend Vaseline® because it has the ideal viscosity). When the time comes for you

Dr. Leah M. Schwartz

to touch her, one of the most important factors in your success will be your confidence and your ability to communicate. Usually the clitoris is partially or completely covered by a foreskin, similar (though smaller) to an uncircumcised penis. As she becomes engorged, more of the head of the clitoris may become exposed. Tell her you're going to touch her vulva now, and gently apply the Vaseline® around the edges of her vulva in decreasing circles until you get to the center. Then, spreading the lips apart, retract the hood of her clitoris. Start light and slow asking as you go if it's all right to increase the pressure or velocity. If she says yes, only do so in very small increments so that you don't override her comfort level. If she finds direct rubbing, no matter how light, too intense, rub her clitoris through the hood. If she finds a really light touch irritating or unbearable, try a nice firm stroke.

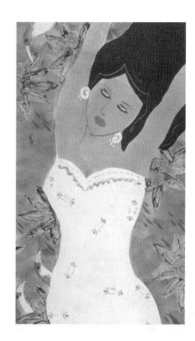

Remember, she is in charge. It's her body and she knows best no matter what you think. If you do this faithfully, she will learn to trust you. Only then will she begin to find a broader range of sensation pleasurable.

As you continue, ask her non-judgmental questions that require simple yes/no answers. For example, "Would you like it a little harder?" If she says yes, rub a little harder and ask again. Continue in this way until she says no, then stick with that pressure for a while. "To the left more?" "Higher?" "Would you like a faster (slower) stroke?" "More lubricant?" This way of communicating is very effective in finding the right spot on the clitoris and discovering which exact amount of pressure, direction or speed feels best. This is the way for you to extract information from her without her having to do anything but give you simple one-word answers.

21

How come the woman in my life won't tell me how to please her?

She may have asked someone before in the past and been disappointed and, for that reason, doesn't want to repeat the experience. Some men are notoriously prideful and defensive whenever they're told they're not doing well enough—particularly when it concerns their sexual performance. This is reinforced by the fact that many women will assure men that what they did was wonderful, when in fact it was no fun at all. It leaves the man convinced he's really adept, when in fact he's pretty lame. When someone finally tries to tell him, his response is "I haven't had any complaints so far."

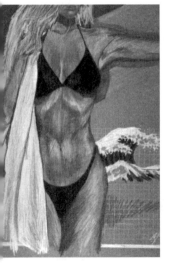

Outside the bedroom she may see how hard it is to get you to do something she wants and figures that in the bedroom, where your ego is really sensitive, she has no chance at all. I suggest that you reassure her that she can say anything to you in the bedroom because your number one goal and desire is that it be the best for her. Invite her on a romantic date and show her how easy it is for her to ask for what she wants. And whatever she asks for—keep your promise! You should be aware that what a woman really wants is to be pleasured beyond anything she could possibly imagine. But because she can only tell you what she can imagine, you have to know that whatever she tells you, she really wants better than that. That's the only way for her to feel overwhelmed and for you to turn into her star.

Dr. Leah M. Schwartz

22 *My partner is sexually inhibited. What can I do to help her come out of her shell?*

Inhibition is a relative matter. To a Victorian prude, your wife might seem to be a shameless hussy. Everyone including you has limitations, and anyone's limitations can be expanded if the person is gently and safely introduced to areas of pleasure they have not previously considered acceptable.

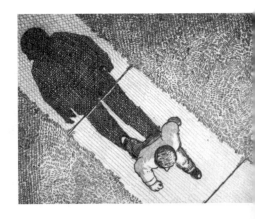

The way to proceed is to do whatever you know causes her pleasure. The moment she indicates in the slightest way that she does not want you to go any further, stop immediately, and do this every time you get involved in a pleasurable cycle.

If you repeat this faithfully without exception, she will come to understand that she can trust you to go no further than she feels comfortable. Be pleased with whatever she permits, enjoy giving her whatever pleasure she will accept and do not make going beyond her limits your goal. She can then relax, confident in your reliability, and allow you to go further and further.

23 My wife and I used to have sex all the time and now we rarely do. What happened?

In the beginning of a relationship, some women are motivated to engage in sex more often because they know that men are looking for women who are enthusiastic about sex. After courting is over, however, they no longer have this same motivation. Similarly, you may be less motivated to be romantic than you were during the dating and courting phase.

Sex is still a fun thing to do, but you have many more things to share in your lives now. If you both want more sex, you are going to have to be more deliberate about it. Talk about it ahead of time, agree upon a time and place, possibly a hotel room, get everything together that you are going to need (drinks, snacks, lubricants, etc.) and take your time.

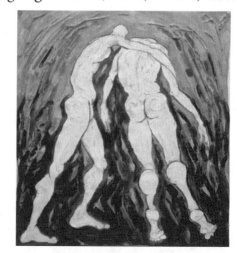

You can achieve more genuine pleasure now that you are familiar with one another's minds and bodies than you could when you were excited about the newness of it all.

Dr. Leah M. Schwartz

24 *I am a man in my sixties and until recently my orgasms were a ten on a scale from one to ten. Now sometimes they are only a seven or eight or even a three. Is it my age? What can I do to bring them back to ten again?*

Orgasms are the release of sexual tension or tumescence. The more tumescence you build, the more tension will be accumulated and the more intensity may accompany its release. Like blowing up a balloon, the more air you get in there, the bigger the bang. The way to build tumescence is the peaking process; five steps forward, one step back, for example.

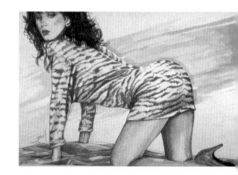

Practice this yourself using a lubricant. Vaseline is best for this because the skin doesn't absorb it and it doesn't evaporate, so you don't have to keep reapplying. Stroke your penis until it feels really good, then back off. Each time you feel the approach of orgasm, stop, bring yourself down slightly and then resume stroking. Repeating this process will build tumescence.

You can continue this for a considerable period of time, taking yourself increasingly higher. When you want to, take yourself over the edge. If you practice this on a regular basis, you will be able to exceed by far the orgasms you used to label a ten. You are never too old to learn how your body works and how to pleasure your partner.

Orgasm

25 *I am a female in my twenties who has never had an orgasm except when masturbating. I am not sexually active. I understand that one needs to really "let go" during sex; however, I was hoping you could give me some pointers on how to reach orgasm. Are there some muscles I am not using or something?*

Yes, your mouth muscles! You are not going to be able to let go with someone who does not know what he is doing. You are going to have to teach him enough so that you can turn your body over to him, knowing you are in good hands.

If he knew as much as you know, he could make you feel a lot better than you can make yourself feel.

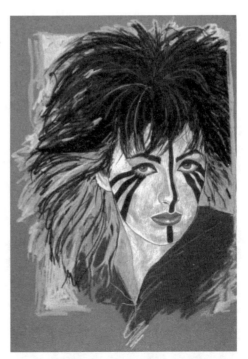

Who Taught You *That*?

26 *I have orgasms with oral sex and masturbation, but I have never had an orgasm during coitus. What can I do to make that happen?*

If you really want to achieve this goal, arrange your body so that the shaft of the man's penis rubs against your clitoris during incursive motions. Chances are, however, that unless your genitals are already well-engorged, it won't work. On the other hand, when you already have perfectly adequate ways of reaching orgasm, why pressure yourself?

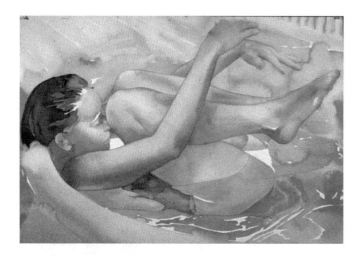

Dr. Leah M. Schwartz

27 *I would like to know more information on how to have an orgasm the "normal way." Do you think I could train myself to have an orgasm during intercourse? I think I had one when I was eighteen, but I am now thirty-eight. Can you offer some suggestions?*

There is no normal way. Whatever works for you is the right and normal way. Have you had orgasms before using methods other than intercourse? If so, that is great. If not, the best way to learn how your body works is to experiment—touching yourself, and giving yourself permission to explore. It is

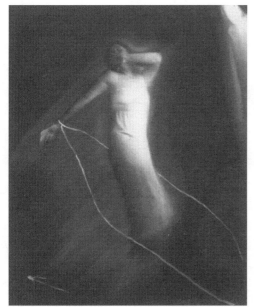

your body, and the only way you can teach a man how to please you is for you to know what pleases you.

How, where, and when to touch yourself is vital. To have an orgasm through intercourse, the best position for a woman is generally on top of the man, because you have control of the action. Also, it is very important that your genitals be engorged, so that your clitoris can maintain contact with his penis. Remember, your most sensitive spot is your clitoris, and, when aroused, it extends towards the opening of the vaginal canal.

28 *Where is the most sensitive spot on the clitoris?*

This is a great question that few people even know to ask. For most women, we think it's our right side, because we are for the most part right-handed. When women masturbate, that's the side they give most attention to. However, most women who have investigated further report that the most sensitive part is the upper left-hand quadrant with the foreskin retracted. However, this is not an absolute, and it would be best for you to experiment and verify this for yourself.

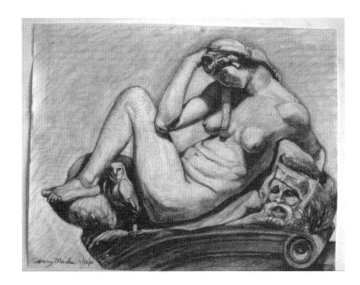

Dr. Leah M. Schwartz

29 If a woman has a big clitoris does she feel more?

No, the size of the clitoris does not determine the sensitivity, but the value judgments you make about your genital parts may affect the pleasure you perceive.

30 Do clitorises come in different sizes?

Yes, just as there are different size penises and breasts, clitoris size also varies. Some are quite prominent and others as so small as to be hard to detect without deliberately retracting the foreskin.

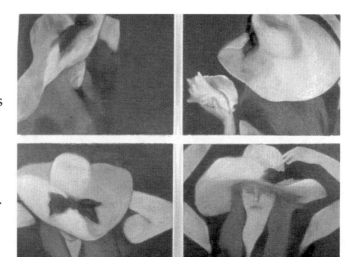

The range is quite large, from a barely discernible protrusion to something resembling a small penis.

31

Is one side of the clitoris more sensitive than the other?

What I have found to be true for myself is that the upper left quadrant of the clitoral head is the most sensitive part of the clitoris. There are always exceptions, but for most women it is the left side.

I would invite any woman to explore for herself with attentive experimentation or, if you are the man, to get into agreement with the woman and, gently retracting the foreskin, stroke her clitoris with a lubricated and manicured fingertip, starting very lightly and gently increasing the pressure. Find out from her which side she finds the most sensitive.

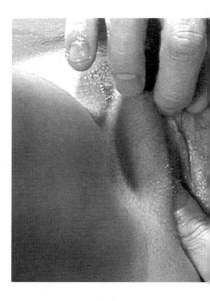

Dr. Leah M. Schwartz

32 *How do you know when you are touching a woman's clitoris that she is enjoying it?*

Remember that you are dealing with the most sensitive area of her body. Not only does the clitoris contain the highest concentration of nerve endings in a woman's body, but it is also covered with an additional layer of skin (the clitoral hood), like the head of an uncircumcised penis. Consequently, it should not be stimulated by direct external contact as with the rest of her skin until her clitoris becomes engorged.

Touch her gently with a well-lubricated finger and keep your attention on her. If, as it seems by your question, your attention is on how well you are doing, your touch will not feel nearly as good to her as it would if you were paying attention to her.

If she is willing to talk to you about this, you should ask her. However, her previous experiences with men's sensitivity about their performance may have made her reluctant to let you know if what you're doing doesn't feel very good. Persist until she feels comfortable telling you.

33 What do a woman's genitals look like when she is turned on?

A woman's genitals, when aroused, can exhibit varying degrees of engorgement from increased blood flow in the area, appearing fuller in the inner and outer lips of the vulva, introitus (or opening to the vagina) and in the head and the shaft of the clitoris.

Depending on the coloration of the genitals when flaccid, or un-aroused, there can be a marked deepening in color. It is also common for some amount of natural lubrication to be present and noticeable.

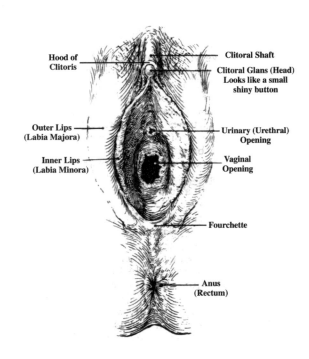

Hood of Clitoris

Clitoral Shaft

Clitoral Glans (Head) Looks like a small shiny button

Outer Lips (Labia Majora)

Urinary (Urethral) Opening

Inner Lips (Labia Minora)

Vaginal Opening

Fourchette

Anus (Rectum)

Dr. Leah M. Schwartz

34

What are some signs that a woman is having an orgasm?

Perineal (the area between the anus and the genitals) contractions are the standard indication of female orgasm. As in the male, they generally occur at eight-second intervals. The average for males is six to nine contractions, and the average for females is nine to twelve, but males and females may experience orgasms lasting for longer periods.

The subsidiary signs of female orgasm include engorgement, darkening of nipples and lips, ridging of abdominal muscles, spreading of fingers and toes, increased respiration, increased heart rate, and flushing in the face and chest, particularly evident in light-skinned individuals. Not all of these will necessarily be present.

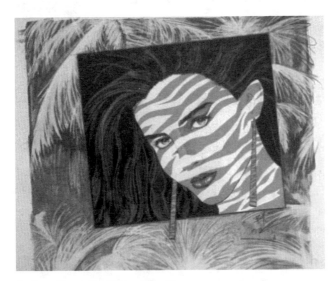

Who Taught You *That*?

35 What can I do to distribute the sensation of my orgasms throughout my body, so that I feel more?

As your pleasure intensifies, you may have a tendency to tighten your musculature, particularly in the pelvic area. This clenching creates a barrier that works to localize the sensation. If you practice reversing this tendency, that is, pushing out and down as you approach orgasm instead of pulling up and in, this will spread the sensation throughout your torso and down your legs. Spreading your fingers and toes will expand the field of pleasurable sensation to your whole body.

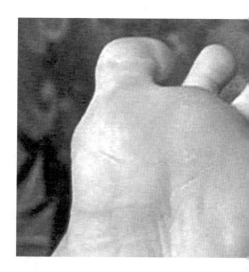

The first few times you practice this, it may result in diminished pleasure because your focus will have shifted from the sensation of the orgasm to reversing the tensing of your muscles. Don't worry about this. You can afford to squander a few orgasms getting it right. Once you learn the technique, it will begin to feel more natural to you, and you won't have to think about it anymore.

Another way to distribute sensation is to recognize that your epidermis is a complete sensing organ, the largest one you have (roughly eighteen square feet), and that your tactile nerves form an interconnected network. If you tickle a baby's feet, its whole body responds.

Dr. Leah M. Schwartz

As we grow up, we learn that our body is made up of separate parts, each with its own name, and this knowledge also teaches us to localize our sensations in those separate parts. With practice, you can learn to reconnect your sensations.

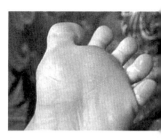

Begin with two highly sensitive areas such as your nipple and your clitoris. Using a lubricant, rub on the areas simultaneously until you begin to feel aroused. Continue to rub on your nipple while taking your hand away from your genitals. Keep your attention on your genitals to see if the sensation in your genitals persists as a result of rubbing on your nipple.

The sensation may be faint at first. When you're certain the sensation is gone, resume rubbing both areas together, this time reversing the process (continue to rub on your genitals while taking your hand away from your nipple). See if you notice a reflection in your nipple this time. When the sensation fades completely, return to rubbing them simultaneously. Keep repeating this cycle until you reach a point where every time your nipple is stimulated, you'll also feel it in your genitals and vice versa.

You can do this with any two areas of your body. If your clitoris and introitus (the opening to your vagina) are well connected, it is easier to achieve orgasm with intercourse. If you have a partner, you can do this to your partner, and your partner can do this to you.

Who Taught You *That?*

36 *How long can an orgasm last?*

This is a question better suited for the *Guinness Book of World Records*. Orgasm is an experience of sensual gratification. Many people think of it as the culmination of the sensual cycle, but in fact, we should learn to think of it more as the beginning. Once a person starts to have regular contractions in the genitals, this pleasurable state can be maintained almost indefinitely if the partner knows what he or she is doing. Asking a question like this is similar to asking how long you expect dinner to last. It could go on for hours and hours as long as you don't make a pig of yourself from the moment you sit down. The analogy is not quite fair because orgasm does not have the same limitations of physical fullness as eating has. The Romans indulged in the practice of periodic vomiting to extend the pleasure of dining.

Your question also implies that duration equates to gratification, which is not the case. Experiment by taking yourself close to the edge—and instead of "going over," keep yourself in this critically delicious state by pausing or applying pressure momentarily. When you decide to take yourself over, instead of going harder and faster, lighten up and slow down and keep on stroking. If you do this several times, you'll discover that what you had considered the end is an intensely pleasurable sensitive condition that can be milked for a prolonged period.

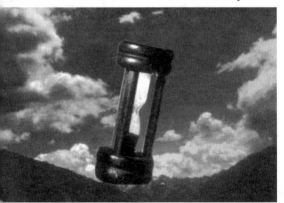

If you're a man, don't think of ejaculation as the end. There is far more pleasure available on the other side.

Dr. Leah M. Schwartz

37

Why have a one-hour orgasm?

Why not?

Why listen to a whole CD instead of just one song?

Or eat Thanksgiving dinner instead of a sandwich?

If pleasure is good, more is better.

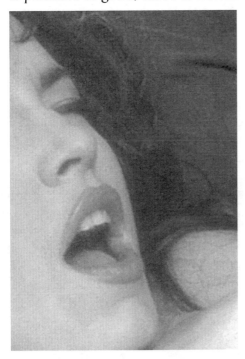

Who Taught You *That?*

38

I enjoy using a vibrator but don't seem to feel quite as much when my boyfriend touches me in the same way. What's wrong?

There is nothing wrong with using a vibrator and as far as I can tell, you have not damaged yourself. What you like about the vibrator is that it allows you the luxury of surrendering to stimulation that does not require a lot of labor to create. The vibrator has accustomed you to intense pressure, but you can still learn to respond to the pleasure of a tender touch. What I recommend is that you start with yourself first, allowing yourself to feel everything from the soft to the intense. You need to be willing to stop comparing every orgasm you have to the orgasms you have with your vibrator and feel what there is to feel when you are touching yourself.

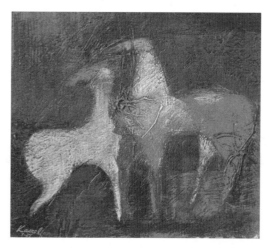

A good way to do this is to purchase one of those rubber hoses from the drugstore that has a showerhead on one end and a socket that fits over the bathtub faucet on the other. Cut off the showerhead, attach the hose to the faucet and adjust the water temperature so that the temperature is tolerable, but pleasant. Lay back in the bathtub (use an inflated plastic pillow for your comfort), open your legs and spread apart your vaginal lips with one hand while directing the flow of water onto your clitoris with the other. Adjust the pressure of the flow by squeezing the end of the hose until the jet is as intense as you like.

Dr. Leah M. Schwartz

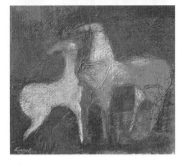

As you become more stimulated, experiment with harder and softer water pressure. Take your time—there is no hurry. Remember, pleasure is the goal, not the rush to go over the edge. Approach the edge as many times as you like, and if you feel like it, go over while continuing to direct the flow onto your clitoris. The brutality of the vibrator prevented you from experiencing a whole world of much subtler sensation—the hose will help you to reset your threshold for sensual response.

If you have a bidet available, you can use it for your investigation in a similar manner. Bidets are very common in Europe and are becoming increasingly popular in American bathrooms. Be sure to check the temperature before you sit on the bidet just as you did with the faucet, and set it so that the temperature is comfortable. Sit on the bidet facing the wall. There is an adjustment on the bidet that allows you to change the pressure from light to intense. Position your clitoris over the jet of water and experiment with the different pressures. The more aroused you become, the wider the range of pressures you will begin to find pleasurable.

Once you have done some of your own investigation, you can begin to teach your lover how to touch you the way that you like to be touched. As with the bidet, the more excited you become the wider the range of pressure you will be able to derive pleasure from.

You may also want to review the answer to Question 35 to reverse the "clenching behavior" you learned with the vibrator. There is far more pleasure available to you than you've been achieving with your very focused and goal-oriented approach.

39

I am a woman and think I am having orgasms in my sleep, sometimes after I have had some drinks. How is this possible?

Dreaming is just as real as when you're awake so that while you're dreaming, anything can happen including things we don't allow to happen while we're awake. If you go to sleep highly tumesced, you're more likely to have an orgasm in your sleep.

You don't need to be touched to have an orgasm. Being touched is a way to increase the tumescence you're already feeling, but if we're tumesced enough, we don't need the stimulation of being touched.

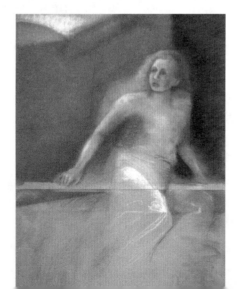

Dr. Leah M. Schwartz

40

How can I help my woman to become multi-orgasmic?

Multiple orgasms are a phenomenon that can go on for as long as the source of stimulation continues.

Producing multiple orgasms in a woman who has not stumbled upon them herself is somewhere between dim and impossible. Multi-orgasmic is only one stage in the evolution of pleasure.

If you put your attention on pleasuring her, she may experience multiple orgasms along the way. If you have that as a specific goal, I doubt that you'll get there.

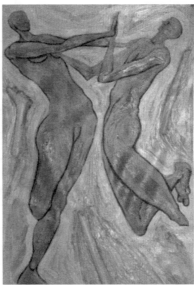

41

What is this flooding thing that happens when my girlfriend touches my G-spot, and how can I make it happen again? It seems to happen when I don't expect it; I would like to make it happen every time. I know it is not urine because we both smelled it to make sure. Where did the liquid come from?

A certain percentage of women report the kind of ejaculation that you describe. Some of them experience it with regularity, others only occasionally. The majority of women never experience it at all, yet they may have extremely pleasurable and satisfying sex lives. The ejaculatory response does not seem to be in and of itself a demonstration of orgasm. It is apparently a physiological side effect that sometimes accompanies pleasure, and there is not complete agreement on its origin.

You say it seems to happen when you don't expect it, but that you'd like to have it happen every time. It would be best if you put your attention back on pleasure and forget about squirting. The more you seek to achieve massive spurting, the less attention you place on your pleasurable responses, which may actually result in less feeling. Consequently, you'll be defeating your own goal.

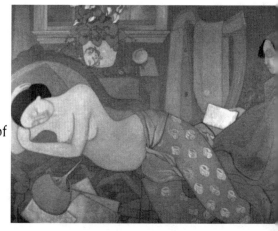

In a society where there is so much pressure to convince our lovers of our sexual adequacy, people are desperate to come up with some kind of proof of their validity. Spurting liquids seems to be a demonstration of sexual value, but the only real validity is how much pleasure you give and take in your sex life.

Dr. Leah M. Schwartz

42

I don't like it when my clitoris is touched directly. When my girlfriend touches me, it has to be on the hood of my clitoris. When I touch her, on the other hand, I am able to do it directly on her clitoris. I would like her to be able to do that to me. What can I do?

Some women are more sensitive in this area than others. The more people expose themselves to specific stimulation, the more they become accustomed to it. There is no reason for you to envy your girlfriend for her particular degree of sensitivity. Where the goal is sensual pleasure, heightened sensitivity is always a good thing. You didn't mention it, but I'd guess that you can touch your own clitoris directly. If you can do this, so could she if you were as confident in her touch as you are in your own.

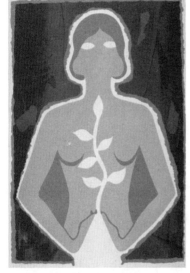

Pay attention to the way you touch yourself. Experiment with different areas, pressures and speeds. You will notice that when you're at the controls, you can tolerate a significant variation in contact. Show your girlfriend how you can touch yourself directly with pleasure. Take her hand in yours, pull back your foreskin and rub on your clitoris using her finger. The more she honors your special preferences, the more confidence she will begin to have in herself, and the more you will be able to relax. A lot of your sensitivity is caused by your apprehension that when someone else is in control, they might do something that would cause you discomfort. Practice with your girlfriend until she knows what you like, and you're sure that she knows how to do it.

Who Taught You *That*?

43 *You say doing the digital thing is the most effective and intense way to satisfy a woman. I really enjoy penetration of my man's penis as well as when he is performing oral sex, or sticking his fingers inside of me. When he does the digital thing, I want his other fingers in me because that is how he gets to my G-spot.*

The clitoris has the highest concentration of nerve endings anywhere in the female body, and women can achieve complete and satisfying orgasms from clitoral contact alone. Many women masturbate exclusively using clitoral stimulation. This does not mean that adding other pleasures like rubbing the clitoris from inside the vaginal canal (the so-called *G-spot*) or rubbing the breasts, vulva, introitus, anus, rectum, or any other part of the body replete with nerve endings will not add to clitoral pleasure.

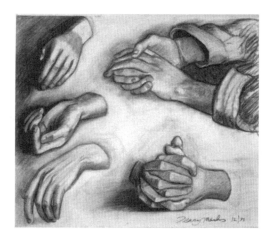

There are no rules or correct methods. Ideas such as this lead to people thinking that they're not doing it right or that there may be something wrong with them. The truth is if pleasure is the goal, whatever works is right. And whatever else you discover is also right.

Dr. Leah M. Schwartz

44 *My fiancé has a large vagina, and I wanted to know if there was anything that I could do to ensure that she had an orgasm every time we had sex.*

The size of her vagina has nothing to do with her orgasms. Her orgasms are generated from her clitoris. You need to learn how to touch her so she will have orgasms every time. You're a good man for caring about the quality of her sex life, but an orgasm every time is a success-oriented goal. You would do better to place your attention on how much pleasure she is having rather than on your success.

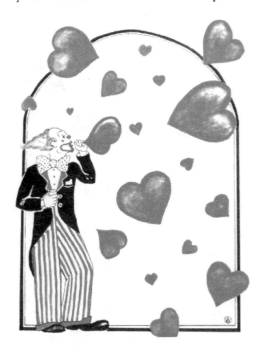

Who Taught You *That?*

Myths and Misconceptions

45 *Is bigger better? Does the size of a man's penis increase the chances for a quicker orgasm in the woman? If a woman's previous lover had a huge penis (ten or more inches), would she become sexually frustrated with her next partner if he were only five to six inches in length? Could the shorter man satisfy her as effectively?*

If reaching orgasm "quicker" is the goal, I have to assume that you are referring to having an orgasm as the result of sexual intercourse. Sexual intercourse is not the

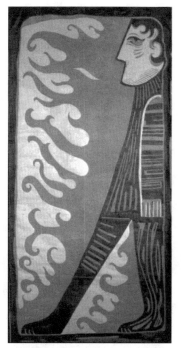

most efficient way for either a man or a woman to have a peak orgasmic experience, so the size of a man's penis has little to do with increasing a woman's chance for a quicker orgasm. If a woman is relying on a penis to produce her orgasm, she will probably feel frustrated with her partner no matter what his size is. Clitoral stimulation is a hit and miss situation if the couple is counting on sexual intercourse to produce orgasm in the female partner.

Your partner can satisfy you by learning how to pleasurably stimulate your clitoris and by engorging your pelvic area. If a woman is engorged, she can feel totally and pleasurably "filled up" with the insertion of as little as the tip of the thumb. Intercourse is more fun for both the woman and the man, regardless of size, when both people are engorged.

Who Taught You *That?*

46 *I am a small woman and my man is large. How can we make love so that I don't get hurt?*

If you want to have intercourse with him, you can. Remember that your vagina is designed to deliver a baby; it is quite elastic. What you need to do is make sure you're sufficiently engorged—that you've been sufficiently stimulated so that your tissues have become saturated with blood and gushy with lubrication. As you become more aroused, the potential for your vagina to accept more penetration increases. Your apprehension about the size of his penis is more likely to dry you up than to lubricate you. Don't hesitate to use a water-soluble artificial lubricant.

You can reassure yourself about the elasticity of your vagina by practicing on yourself, introducing several fingers or your whole hand into your vaginal canal. Talk to your man about your concerns. He could gently massage the opening to your vagina with a couple of his fingers, pressing against the walls with semi-circular motions, gradually relaxing the circular muscle at the opening of your vaginal canal, before inserting his penis.

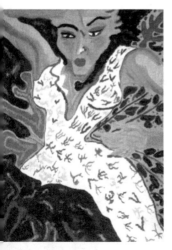

Your concerns about his size may also be causing you to defensively pull up and in, which foreshortens your vagina. If you push down and out, your vaginal canal will lengthen and your cervix will be pulled out of line of his stroke, so that you can accept the head of his penis into the pocket that lies behind your cervix. Pressure in this area can be quite pleasurable. Staying in communication with him and having him follow your instructions will put you in control of the situation and will allay your fears of being assaulted. Don't do anything until you're ready, and only do as much as you enjoy doing.

Dr. Leah M. Schwartz

47 Can men have multiple orgasms?

Yes, they can. Most men are heavily committed to the idea that ejaculation signals the end of their sexual cycle. They complain that the post-ejaculatory penis is too sensitive to enjoy further stroking. "Too sensitive" means extremely sensitive, and this is an ideal condition for wonderful pleasurable experiences if the partner is willing to slow down and lighten up.

Most people are committed to harder and faster action as they approach ejaculation. To reverse this trend, we must be willing to explore those vast areas of untapped pleasures that lie beyond ejaculation.

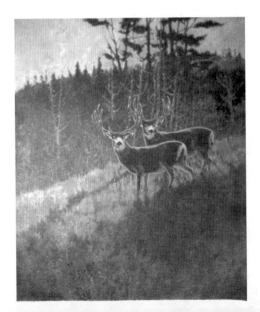

Who Taught You *That*?

48
Does abstinence shorten the amount of time it takes for a man to reach orgasm?

In some men, scarcity of sex would increase excitement causing the man to ejaculate sooner, sometimes even before insertion. However, there is no absolute correlation between frequency of sexual activity and the speed of climax.

49
I am a man and my orgasms seem to be weak with not much fluid coming out. What is that about?

Although many men evaluate their sexual performance in such terms, there is no absolute relationship between the amount of ejaculate and the intensity of orgasm.

A man can ejaculate a cup full and feel barely anything or have his head ripped off and hardly spurt at all. Get back into your body, and find what feels right to you and go from there.

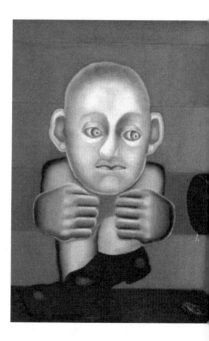

Dr. Leah M. Schwartz

50

How can I last longer than two minutes?

In general, questions about men lasting longer are based on the commonly held belief that intercourse is the best way to achieve sexual satisfaction or simultaneous orgasm. This is not true. For women, the highest concentration of nerve endings, and consequently the most sensitive part of their anatomy, is in the clitoris, not in the lining of the vagina. The highest concentration of nerve endings in a man's body is in the head of the penis.

For both men and women, the greatest pleasure comes from total effect. In other words, the most satisfying feelings come from putting all your attention on your sensation. When a man is trying to produce more pleasure for a woman by trying to avoid his own pleasure, he is doing neither. The way to produce the most pleasure for your lover is to put all of your attention on her, which is impossible if you're trying to control your own pleasurable responses.

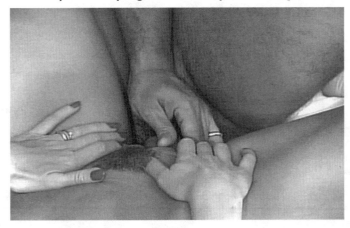

If you will learn how to manually pleasure your woman's clitoris, you can produce far more pleasure for her than you can by pumping her vagina, even if you're able to arrange your body so that your penis is in contact with her clitoris. If you learn to gratify her manually, she won't care how long or short a time you take gratifying yourself.

Who Taught You *That?*

51

How come many men wake up with erections in the morning and think it means it is time to make love?

Many men are conditioned to believe that having a hard penis means they ought to do something with it or about it. This is another myth. Males experience erections whether there's an aroused female around or not. They experience erections in response to contact or pressure in the genital region.

It is common for pressure from a full bladder to trigger an erection in a waking male, but this does not necessarily mean he should have sex. It probably means he should urinate. Many men in our culture consider their sensuality as external validation of their masculinity and feel they should cash in on every erection.

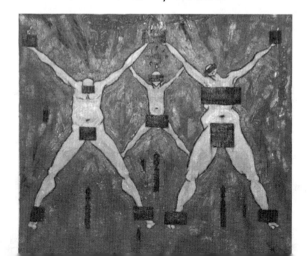

Dr. Leah M. Schwartz

52 *Is it true that men reach their sexual peak at eighteen and women at thirty-five?*

This question implies that men and women of these ages are ideal lovers. When it comes to questions about our biology, it is important to remember that we are big-brained creatures. Our sensual relationships are not simply a response to drives. It is true that at certain times of the month, the year or our lives, we may be more predisposed (in a biochemical sense) to sexing than at other times, but this certainly doesn't mean that we go out and "do it." The fact is that most of our sexing is done for social reasons. We sex when, where and with whom we choose based on decisions made in accordance with the practices and prejudices of the society in which we live.

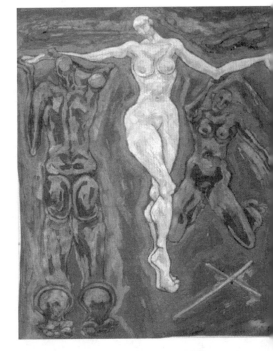

Regardless of the biological profile, a thirty-five year old woman in our society rarely finds an eighteen year old an appropriate mate, and eighteen year old guys don't often drool after women twice their age. Women offer attractiveness, which in our society is heavily associated with youth, whereas men offer their productivity, which is more likely to peak in older, well-established males.

Who Taught You *That*?

53

As a woman, what can I do to increase my sexual drive?

What makes this a difficult question to answer is that you as with so many other women think that there is a certain feeling you need to have in order to have sex, certain sensations that you want to feel in your body. But the best way to increase your sexual desire is to start with your brain. What I mean by this is that most of us will only "give in" to our desires once we begin to have certain feelings in our body.

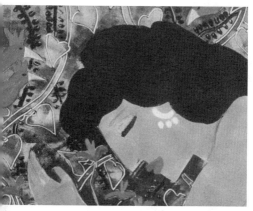

If you allow yourself to think wonderful sexual thoughts about your lover such as how good he smells, how good he looks, how much you like the way it feels when he caresses you, touches you in that special way, you will start to feel turned on, which is natural and healthy. Knowing and anticipating a good and fun time can make you feel excited as well. Plan deliberate sex dates. You can be deliberate about your sexual desire. You do not have to wait for the turn-on fairy. Once you see that you are in charge of your turn-on, you will feel freed, knowing you can have great sex anytime you want.

The viewpoint in our society is that you have to be "in the mood" before you can want to have sex, but you can create those feelings in yourself through your deliberate thoughts and actions.

Dr. Leah M. Schwartz

54

How can I improve my sex life?

Begin by having it right the way it is. Things go from good to better. You cannot get to better from bad without going through good. Going from good, you can increase the quality, the quantity or both. Sex is a form of communication. It is the giving and receiving of pleasure. You can only truly provide your partner with the most pleasure possible if you are enjoying what you are doing. Do only those things you want to do and only for as long as you want to do them.

Many people cling to the idea that sex is doing what comes naturally, but no one thinks that about their tennis game or playing the piano. People who wish to get better at these activities understand that they need to practice. The more talented they are, the more they practice. If you want to improve your sex life, make the decision to do something about it.

Find yourself a partner you enjoy being with and investigate pleasuring one another. Set up deliberate dates for sensual research and talk to your lover about what you like and find out from them what they like. As you continue these training sessions, you'll become more and more familiar with one another's bodies and how to best please one another. If you continue diligently, you'll find you get better and better at giving and receiving pleasure.

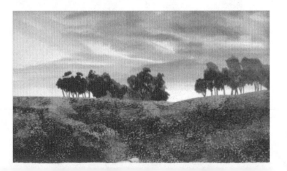

Who Taught You *That*?

55 How often should we have sex?

There is no right amount. Many people are needlessly concerned about frequency, when the real answer is *whenever you want to*, which is probably what you are already doing. If you do not think you are getting enough, you could talk it over with your partner. If one of you wants to do it more than the other, take care of it by agreeing that one of you will help the other achieve the pleasure they want or that you will take care of yourself when your partner is not particularly interested.

Nobody is responsible for your sex life but you.

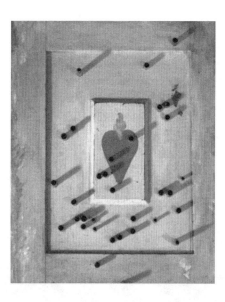

56 How long should our lovemaking last?

If reproduction is the goal, no longer than the first ejaculation.

If the goal is enjoyment, as long as the pleasure continues.

Dr. Leah M. Schwartz

57 *I want to improve my sex life, but my husband thinks I am crazy. Why?*

I'm afraid you may have brought this on yourself. You may have given him the idea over the course of your marriage that everything was just hunky-dory. Now you're trying to change that conception, and it doesn't jibe with what you've been telling him. Everything's been wonderful up to now, and now you want to improve it? No wonder he thinks you're crazy.

For many men, getting it up, getting it in and having an orgasm is the very definition of good sex. Assuming it's the same for the woman is an opinion that can't ever change as long as we continue to give the impression that it's true.

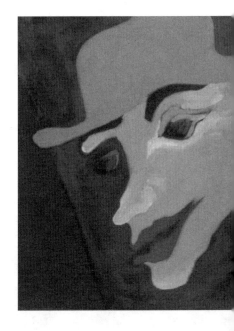

Men validate themselves very heavily on their ability to gratify women. One way a woman can gain a man's attention and favor is by assuring him that he's winning with her sexually. If you want to communicate with your husband about this issue, recognize how important winning is for him, and begin your communication by focusing on the things he's doing right. Enthusiastically acknowledge when he succeeds. People like to win, and he will enjoy a game that he continually improves at.

Who Taught You *That*?

58

How come when some people fight they want to have sex right afterwards?

Not all people want to have sex after a fight. There is a widespread viewpoint that there are occasions in a man-woman relationship when it is sex or fight time. This is based on the fact that both sexing and fighting are ways to detumesce.

Tumescence refers to a buildup of energy. Some people express tumescence by becoming irritable, which can then lead to arguing or fighting. If tumescence is running high, sometimes people will fight because they are unwilling to think about the sex it would take to bring them down. Consequently, they will start a fight to release some of the tumescence. Then, when the pressure has been lowered enough for them to confront their sensual feelings, they'll kiss and make up.

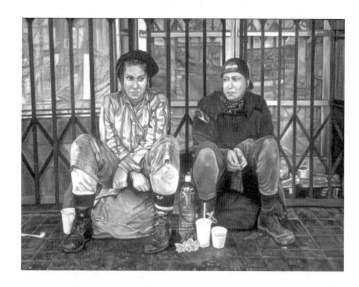

Dr. Leah M. Schwartz

59 *Is it true that if a woman's tongue is cold, she has just had an orgasm?*

It is true that cool extremities occur when blood concentrates in the pelvic area during tumescence. However, it's certainly not a guarantee of a woman's orgasm.

60 *Why do women fake their orgasms?*

Women fake orgasms as a manipulative technique. Their motives for faking orgasm vary. Sometimes they do it to get approval, sometimes to build up the ego of the man they're with, sometimes to end a tiresome sex act—there's no single one reason. However, faking is deception and will eventually poison the relationship.

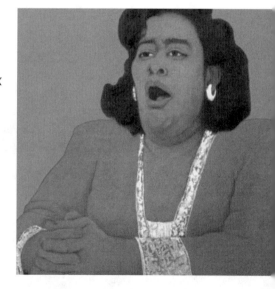

Who Taught You *That?*

61 *How did women learn to fake their orgasms?*

From trying to please their men. Most women realize that men place a high value on their ability to pleasure women. Letting a man know that he hasn't measured up can rapidly turn into a nasty confrontation, and faking is a convenient way to end a sexual cycle with a man who clearly has no idea what he is doing.

62 *Why do women still fake orgasms?*

Sexually naïve women have only two choices when they don't climax and are lucky enough to be asked—either to lie or to tell the truth. "I didn't have an orgasm" is not politically correct. Some men are so egocentrically involved in performance that women don't want to deal with the hassles they'd evoke if they told the truth. Consequently, for the sake of avoiding conflict, it's often still safer to lie.

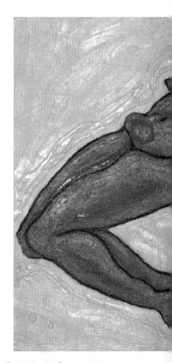

Dr. Leah M. Schwartz

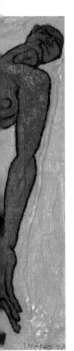

63 *Is there anything wrong with a woman faking an orgasm every once in a while?*

It depends on your goal. If you want to brush the guy off, it may be a reasonable thing to do. If you're interested in forging a long-term relationship with him, starting off with a lie is no way to do it. Moreover, lying also provides him with false information about how to please you.

64 *Should a woman tell a man she has been faking her orgasms?*

It depends on the goal. If the goal is to make a friend of this person, then yes, she should tell him. If the goal is to manipulate him, then she should keep the matter to herself. A woman should not tell a man she has been faking her orgasms unless she intends to correct the situation. Otherwise, it could blow up in her face.

65

If you choose to tell your man that you have been faking your orgasms, what should you say?

Just tell him the truth. "I have not been orgasming well enough." "What about all those orgasms you had last week?" "Yeah, that's the problem—I was faking it. But I've found a way to improve our sex life, and I thought it was important to start with the truth."

There is no lie you can tell that justifies not telling the truth—it is a matter of morality. It is morally wrong to lie to your friends, and in this day and age, you shouldn't be having sex with someone who isn't your friend. If you really are friends and you orgasm so little that you feel you must fake it, you have an obligation to one another, yourselves and to the relationship to increase your orgasmic index.

(See the answer to questions 20 and 75 to get yourself started.)

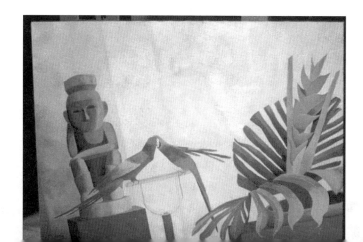

Dr. Leah M. Schwartz

66

Do you think that some men believe that they know everything there is to know about pleasing a woman, or is it that they don't care?

Some men care about pleasing women not so much for the sake of the woman as for the validation of their own prowess. Hence the standard joke, "Was it good for you, honey?"

Because women have a tendency to provide positive feedback regardless of the quality of the experience, men have no reliable standards by which to evaluate their performance.

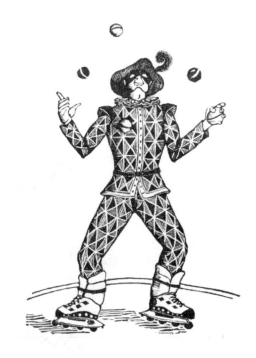

67 *I have heard a lot about Kegal exercises. Do they really help to make sex better for men and for women?*

I would not categorically deny that doing Kegals would have the effect of improving sensual pleasure. It is probable that any method which directs your attention to your genitals and exercises the surrounding musculature would bring blood to the genital area and effectually engorge the tissue. Kegals specifically repeatedly clench the opening to the vaginal canal. This has the effect of gripping the base of an inserted penis and permitting the woman and man to feel the incursive stroking of the penis at the opening to the vagina.

A more effective means would be to apply the pushout method, which would provide contact for the entire length of the penis and the vagina.

(See the answers to Questions 9 and 35 for information on pushouts).

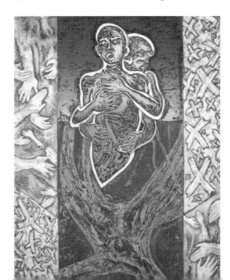

Dr. Leah M. Schwartz

68 Why is talking about sex still considered taboo?

All social rules are prohibitions against behaviors that people were engaging in before the rules came along. In every social system people have been attracted to sexual activity. Consequently, every social order that we know of has some regulations designed to limit when, where, how and with whom sexual activity including the discussion of such may take place.

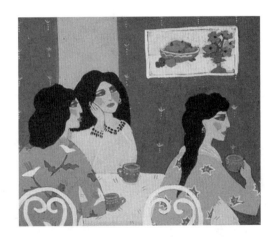

Our society underwent a so-called sexual revolution in the latter part of the last century. When a society experiences a liberation of social inhibitions, the more conservative members of the culture get upset, protesting that society has taken a turn for the worse. In order to pacify this disgruntled group, there's a corresponding swing toward re-establishing the social prohibitions.

The pendulum swings both ways, but it never swings as far back as it was before it swung forward. It is certainly easier for people to talk about sex now than it was in the fifties, but inhibitions still remain.

Who Taught You *That*?

Getting In The Mood

69

My wife is very shy, and I am trying new ways of making love. How do I help her to get over her fears?

How did you approach the subject of sex with her in the beginning? Has she always been shy about sex? What does she like about sex? You cannot make anyone do anything they do not want to do. Make it safe for her to tell you what she likes, and be very receptive to her requests. Make if fun for her.

Take her out on a romantic date, and treat her to her favorite food, favorite drink, favorite music, and favorite flowers. Seeing the time you put into making the date special for her will make her feel good, and will also help her to understand that enjoying herself is okay. If what you're doing to your wife feels good to her, she'll want to experience more of it. If it doesn't, she won't.

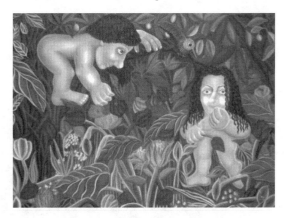

Who Taught You *That*?

70 *How can I get my mate to relax? Overexcitement and worry is sure killing the mood.*

The best way is for you to get your mate to tell you what he or she is overexcited or worried about. If you really, actively listen to what your mate is saying, it will help them to get out of their head and back into their body.

Your mate will be able to relax to the extent that he or she has confidence that you are ready to help them work through it.

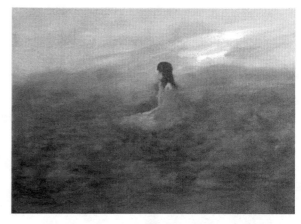

Dr. Leah M. Schwartz

71

What are some things that I can do to stimulate my husband in bed?

Enjoy his being there and let him know how much you do. Let him know what you're going to do before you do it, so there is no surprise. Start touching him far away from his genitals—his hands or his feet. Let him know there's nothing he needs to do.

Use a comfortable, friendly touch, and as he responds, you can move slowly toward his crotch area. Continually reassure him how much you're enjoying yourself—he is sure to respond.

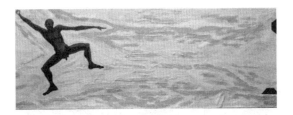

Who Taught You *That?*

72

I have been with my boyfriend for three years now. Our sexual relationship was thrilling during the first year and a half, but now it is dwindling on both sides. I would love some advice on how to rejuvenate it.

You are waiting for what we call the "Turn-on Fairy." There is no such thing. In the initial stages of a relationship, sex is brand new and, as with anything new, it can get old. When you buy a new house or a new car, you feel excited. To sustain those initial feelings of excitement, you have to be deliberate about doing the maintenance to keep that house or that car looking new and beautiful. Your sexual relationship is the same way. Being deliberate means trying new things with each other.

The greatest aphrodisiac is anticipation. Setting up a sex date is a good way to revive those old feelings in your relationship. His part is just to follow your instructions and be enthusiastic about what you set up. Practice, practice, practice. That's the key.

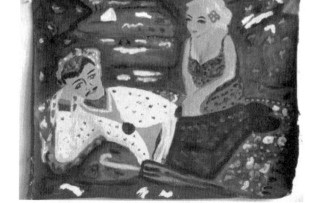

Dr. Leah M. Schwartz

73

How can we get in the mood at the same time?

Communicate with one another. Be honest about how aroused you feel. You can have more fun starting from genuine flat than from a phony turn-on. Be willing to admit what you are willing to do and what you are unwilling to do, with the understanding that once you get started, you could change your mind in either direction. Most of us are waiting for the "Turn-on Fairy." Well, there isn't one.

The good news is that you can make love anytime if you'll just be deliberate. If you'll just start at flat or a low level of turn-on, you can end up in the mood that you were looking for. Set up dates with each other. Tell each other what you find pleasurable about one another, touch each other in ways that feel good, and acknowledge to one another the fun you are having.

You can start at flat and do what feels good and before you know it, you will feel like a towering inferno. Saying sensual things to each other, thinking about being touched, talking about memories of past pleasures or fantasies of future ones, are all arousing.

The mind is the most powerful sexual organ.

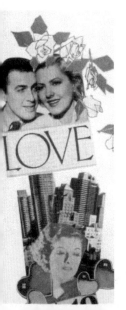

Who Taught You *That?*

74

As much as we enjoy making love, why don't we do it more often?

Scheduling time together these days is tough enough, without having to wait for passion to walk in the door at the same time.

Rather than making the agreement that you won't have sex until you both want to, why not make an agreement to have sex when the time becomes available? If only one of you is in the mood then, or even if neither of you is, you can *still do it* and both enjoy it. Neither one of you has to be in the mood necessarily; you just have to want to.

If people only had sex when they were both in the mood, world population would drastically fall. Animals engage in sex when the strongest one wants to. Human beings engage in sex when they both agree there's nothing better to do. Being in the mood has nothing to do with it.

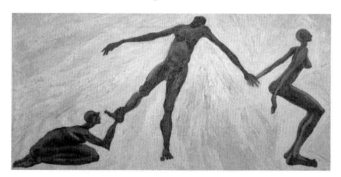

Dr. Leah M. Schwartz

75

How do I tell my lover what I want in the bedroom?

Factoring in the experience and attentiveness of your lover, you are still going to need to be as direct as possible to get him or her to do what you know would pleasure you. If talking doesn't get it across, you may actually have to show your lover what you want—take their hand in your hand and touch yourself with it so that they can feel what areas, degree of pressure, and velocity please you most.

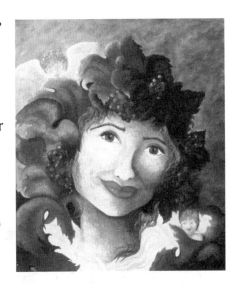

Some people are quite sensitive when it comes to criticism of their sexual performance. Thus, it would be best to get your lover's agreement in advance before investing the time and effort in such an exercise. Be pleased with them for being with you. Express approval for the things that you like and suggest ways to make them even better. Give them big wins when they move in that direction. Keep the session short; tell them you enjoyed it, and that you'd like to do it again sometime.

Who Taught You *That?*

76

How can you have the most fun with a sensual experience?

You can have the most enjoyment by including the three time periods—future, present and past. Think about it before it happens, enjoy anticipating what's going to happen, enjoy preparing for it and getting ready, enjoy it while it's happening and communicate your pleasure.

When it's over, enjoy remembering it and reminiscing about it.

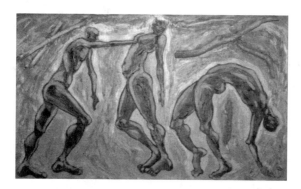

Dr. Leah M. Schwartz

77 *What about fantasy?*

If you communicate those fantasies, it can enhance the turn-on in your relationship. Fantasies are those things we enjoy conceptually but not necessarily in reality. Assure one another that having a fantasy does not necessarily mean that you actually want to do such things. That will make it safer to expose intimate conceptions that you have enjoyed.

Fantasizing during sex about real or imaginary experiences doesn't mean you'd prefer them to the experience you're having. It is like spice—not a very good diet, but it sure adds flavor to the meal.

Who Taught You *That?*

78

Why is foreplay so important to women?

The very idea of foreplay is the pleasure that comes before. Before what? In our society, the 'what' means intercourse. This concept is goal-oriented. Sensuality is oriented around pleasure, which is not concerned with attainment but with the way it feels now.

What we call foreplay is really just having fun with one another. The rush to get off is fostered by an attitude of scarcity—get it while you can. But if it feels good, why rush it?

Just as you would savor a seven-course meal, so should you with a sensual experience. In times of feast or famine, it is best to move slowly.

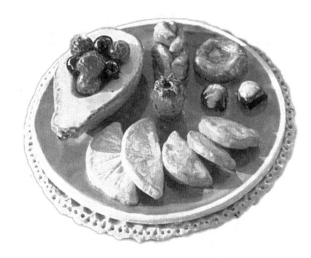

Dr. Leah M. Schwartz

79

How do you establish trust in the bedroom?

You keep your agreements with each other and respond (honestly) to each other's requests for pleasure. If the request is not attractive, just say so. Do not do what you do not want to do. It could lead to your expecting something in return. Trust in or out of the bedroom depends on predictability.

When someone says they trust you, it means they are counting on you to behave in a certain way. If you want to appear trustworthy, do those things that you have led them to expect you to do. Be reliable.

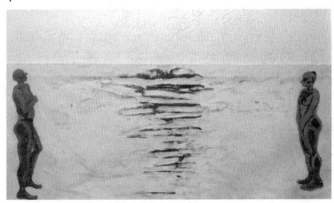

Who Taught You *That*?

80 *How come my husband doesn't want to have sex sometimes?*

No one wants to make love all the time any more than people want to eat or dance all the time. Men don't want to make love when they are not turned on. Not all men have a problem with performance anxiety, but many certainly do. The reason that many men experience performance anxiety is because we live in a production-oriented society where erections equate to achievement.

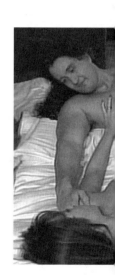

An erection is a physiological response to something or someone sexually attractive, just as salivation is a response to delicious food. Men who think they are responsible for producing their own erections may find themselves incapable of doing so on one occasion when it seemed quite easy on another. Having had this experience, they may fear a repetition the next time around and since fear is such a poor aphrodisiac, they may well have trouble again thus creating a cycle of failure.

No wonder men experience such anxiety when they think that having sex requires an erection. This is far from true. In fact, it's possible to experience all kinds of pleasure without a hard penis. The greatest pleasure available to a man is in the gratification of his woman. He could pleasure her orally or manually and produce far greater pleasure than he could with a hard penis.

Dr. Leah M. Schwartz

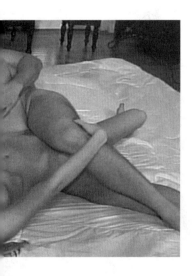

Sensuality is distinct from sexuality. The goal of sexuality is insertion and impregnation. A hard, ejaculating penis is best for this because it deposits the sperm deep within the vagina. The goal of sensuality is pleasure, the stimulation of the tactile receptors distributed throughout the epidermis and body cavities. These can be pleasured orally and manually with far more sensitivity and dexterity than could ever be achieved with a hard penis.

If you are friendly enough with your lover, penetration can be achieved (if desired) with a completely soft penis. All that's required is sufficient lubrication, natural or applied, and the comfortable arrangement of your bodies so that your crotches are up against one another in such a way that his penis can be slipped between your vaginal lips and into your introitus. You can enjoy some wonderful squishy intercourse this way that may be surprisingly pleasurable for both of you, particularly if you're accustomed to a hard penis.

Who Taught You *That*?

81

Why do women so often have to initiate sex? It wasn't always like that.

In our society these days, it's not acceptable if it is not the woman's idea. Because the social and sexual mores of our society are changing so fast, sensitive men want to stand back until they're sure the woman wants to be involved. It used to be romantic to steal a kiss...now it's sexual harassment.

A wise man these days and times is best off asking on each step, and on most steps waiting for her to initiate.

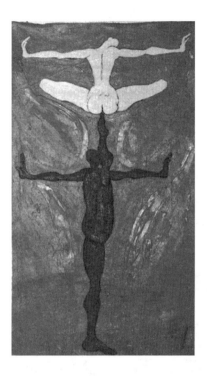

Dr. Leah M. Schwartz

82 What can I do to help her enjoy performing oral sex more than she does?

Many women are reticent to get involved with a penis for fear that once they start, they will become obligated to produce an ejaculation. If you could assure her that she is free to limit her contact with your penis to as little or as much as she chooses, she'd be more willing to begin a cycle.

There is a position where the couple lies facing each other with their heads pointing in opposite directions. The man manually or orally pleasures the woman's vulva, predominately the clitoris, bringing her closer to orgasm then pulling away, so that she is in a state of high arousal before she even has contact with his penis. She can then begin to enjoy his penis with her hands or mouth in whatever ways she finds pleasurable.

As you approach your orgasm, continue to stimulate her genitals. If you make sure that she is aroused before involving her with your penis, stroking your penis will become an additional pleasure for her.

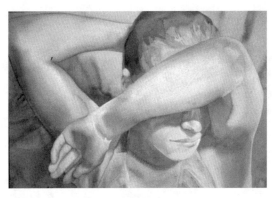

Who Taught You *That*?

83
Why does my desire to watch her touch herself offend or embarrass her?

A woman being conspicuously turned on titillates most men. The embarrassment doesn't come from her touching herself. The embarrassment comes from you wanting her to make a show of her arousal.

Consequently, she may be feeling pressure to display more arousal than she actually feels.

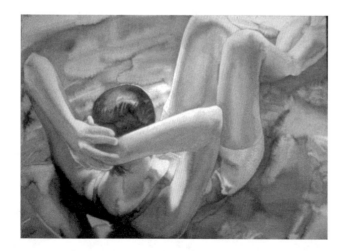

Dr. Leah M. Schwartz

The Sexual Experience

84

How come men and women often will say no to sex?

The only reason to refuse an offer of sex is fear of loss. Even though sex is reputed to be one of the most fun activities that people can experience, there are many occasions when the prospect looks like a loser. The loss may be as obvious as a shortage of time, which would cause them to lose the opportunity to do something else they consider more important or pressing, or as personal as a fear that they will have to perform beyond their level of desire.

Nobody really refuses pleasure; they are refusing the loss they fear would result if they accepted. If you can guarantee them that whatever loss they imagine will definitely not occur (for example, in a case where time is short, that the obligation will definitely be satisfied) or that they won't have to perform at all, just lie back and enjoy, then their resistance can be handled.

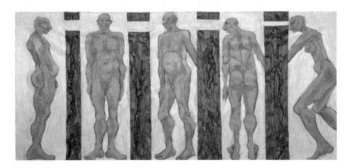

Dr. Leah M. Schwartz

85

What if my mate wants to do something weird and kinky and I don't?

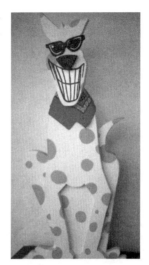

Don't do anything you don't want to do. However, don't dismiss experiences too quickly just because they are beyond what you have found acceptable up to now. Be at least willing to talk about them, reserving for yourself the right to refuse.

If you trust your mate, and if what is proposed is something that other people seem to find pleasure in, you might check it out to see if there is potential for you. Even if you don't discover it the first time, you might give it one more chance before you dismiss it completely. As with food, some tastes are acquired.

Who Taught You *That*?

86 *What is the difference between erotic and sensual?*

Erotic refers to the violation of minor social rules, like showing cleavage or talking dirty, or behaving in ways that society considers naughty or nasty. Erotic has more to do with outside influences, such as doing it in public, doing it in an airplane, or using sex toys. All of this is fine, as long as it is legal.

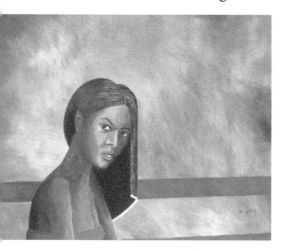

Sensuality refers to the pleasurable stimulation of our sensory receptors. Sensual is all about feeling, feeling each sensation, stroke by stroke. Ways to accomplish this might include increasing the duration or amount of time you let yourself have pleasure, or increasing the intensity of what you feel. It is all about feeling moment to moment, touching the nerve endings in ways that make us feel good. It is all about sensations.

Dr. Leah M. Schwartz

87

What things can I use in my house for sensual pleasure?

Believe it or not, you can use almost anything, within reason. That's because your whole life experience is made up of sensual perceptions and the ideas that you have about those perceptions.

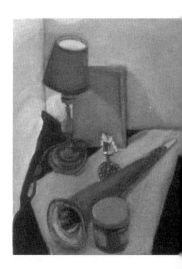

Because you experience all the things in your house through sight, sound, smell, touch, or taste, the conceptual thoughts you have about them are for the most part value judgments. Thus, the pleasure you experience in your life is due to positive judgments associated with your perceptions. If you bring a bunch of flowers into your living room, arrange them in a vase, sit back and say "Oh, how lovely," you have added significantly to the pleasure in your life.

Look around your house and see how you feel about all the things that are there. If you notice anything that could be made to feel better, set about accomplishing it. Clean it, polish it, paint it, cover it, or rearrange it. The idea is to find it good, but to make it better. Cover that scratchy old upholstery with something that feels good on your skin. Add more light, color, and fragrance to your rooms. Introduce music that you like into your environment—turn what you eat and drink into a pleasurable experience as well as a nutritional one. If there's something you dislike, get rid of it. Give it to someone else, and replace it with something you like.

If you are responsible for serving you own sensual preferences, you can make your own life more pleasurable, and the pleasure you feel will be reflected in the ways in which you relate with the world and with other people.

Who Taught You *That*?

88 How many spots are there for pleasure?

There is no precise number of "spots." Traditionally, many writers on sexuality referred to the *erogenous* zones. These were areas of the body that were considered to be more sensitive, with a greater number of nerve endings, such as the lips, nipples, back of the neck, insides of arms and legs, and genitals.

But the human epidermis is covered with nerve endings. Consequently, any area is capable of being pleasured if stimulated in an agreeable manner. It is not nearly as important where you rub as how. The most important element in caressing your lover is the attention you give to him or her.

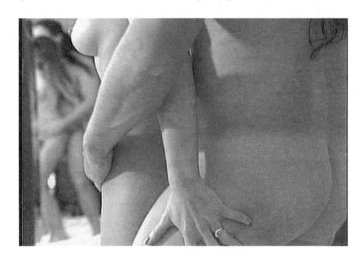

Dr. Leah M. Schwartz

89

Do men and women reach orgasm the same way?

Both men and women can experience pleasurable sensations and involuntary contractions by having their homologous genital parts stimulated, those being the head of the penis in the man and the head of the clitoris in the woman. Masters and Johnson report that on average men experience six to nine contractions per orgasm and woman nine to twelve.

While an upper limit has not been established, it has been documented that both women and men can experience orgasm well beyond the reported averages. Also, ejaculation usually accompanies orgasm in a man giving him the sensation of fluid being expelled through his penis at the moment of orgasm.

Some women have the same sensation of ejaculating a large amount of fluid during orgasm. However, the expulsion of ejaculate is not necessary for either a man or a woman to experience orgasm.

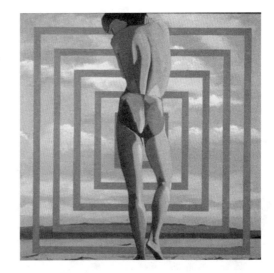

90 Is there a right amount of engorgement and lubrication?

The right amount of lubrication is enough to be able to rub areas of the body continuously with no danger of abrasion. If lubrication seems insufficient, artificial lubricants are readily available. Of these, water-soluble lubricants are best applied to internal cavities. Petroleum-based lubricants like Vaseline® are to be used only for surface stimulation since they are not absorbed by the skin and don't evaporate. Consequently, the caressing of the nerve endings in the skin does not have to be interrupted to apply extra lubrication.

The "right" amount of engorgement for both men and women is whatever amount is produced by pleasurable stimulation of the genitals or other areas. Engorgement is produced by a concentration of blood. In order to engorge the genitals, pressure in a stroking, milking motion or sucking will concentrate increasing amounts of blood there. Other areas such as breasts, lips, etc. may be similarly engorged. Engorgement increases the sensitivity of the nerve endings in the engorged areas.

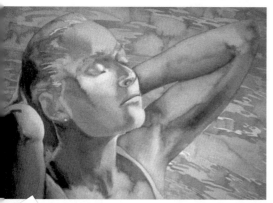

Female lubrication and male engorgement are physiological conditions that are commonly considered necessary for intercourse and, consequently, are common areas of questions in an intercourse-oriented society such as ours in which other forms of sensual pleasuring are called foreplay (necking, petting, etc.) as distinguished from "going all the way" or "the real thing." Women's engorgement is largely overlooked, and this lack of attention is a serious detriment to female pleasure.

Dr. Leah M. Schwartz

91

What is the average penetration time before male and female orgasm?

Statistical averages are plentiful in literature on sex, but they are based on polling limited numbers of people, and responders to the questions are likely to lie, particularly when the questions are about something as sensitive as their sex lives. Penetration in and of itself is not a measure of either male or female orgasm or pleasure.

If what you're doing feels good, there's no reason to hurry, and if it doesn't feel good, you're not going to achieve orgasm by persisting. In other words, forget average times and follow your own instincts.

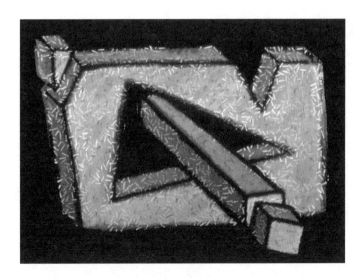

Who Taught You *That*?

92 *Is there another spot on a man besides the obvious place to give him pleasure?*

The epidermis (skin) is the largest sensing organ we have. It is roughly eighteen square feet of sensitive area, any part of which may be stimulated to cause pleasure.

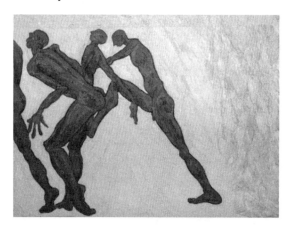

Dr. Leah M. Schwartz

93

How can I improve the pleasuring of my man's penis?

The penis does not end with the pubic hair, but continues all the way to the anus. This can be clearly felt when the penis is erect. The *perineum* is between his scrotum and anus. Using lubricant, stroke his penis with one hand while simultaneously stroking the perineum in the same direction with the other hand. That way you can stroke the whole

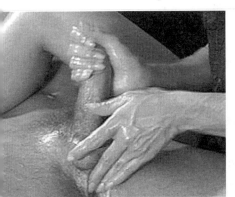

length of his penis using both of your hands. Many women feel the up stroke with their hand and not necessarily the down stroke. Take your time to feel every increment of each stroke in either direction. The more that you feel, the more he will feel. Stay in communication with him, particularly when you begin, and get feedback from him as to what feels best.

Another good spot to stimulate is the coronal ridge of the head of his penis, the part of the head closest to his body that flares out some before the shaft begins. This is a particularly sensitive part of the head. It would be best to lighten up some as you stroke, especially on an uncircumcised penis. There's a notch in the center of the underside of the coronal ridge, which is highly receptive to stimulation. With your hand around his penis so that your thumb is on the underside, rub the notch up and down with the ball of your thumb. Start gently and increase the pressure in small increments.

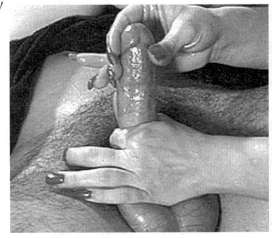

Paying attention to these areas will add to your own enjoyment as well as his.

Who Taught You *That*?

94 *Does the "G-spot" exist and, if so, where is it?*

There is no general agreement among anatomists or neurologists on the existence of the *G-spot*. Dr. Grafenberg first reported the *G-spot* over 50 years ago. Consequently, there has been plenty of time for other researchers to confirm his findings. No one has been able to confirm the existence of the G-spot. The press is continually looking for sensational articles about sensuality, and someone periodically exhumes the *G-spot* and creates some hoopla about it, but as far as modern science is concerned, the *G-spot* is more myth than fact.

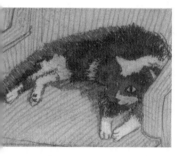

There are many sensitive spots inside the vagina including an area behind the clitoris. This spot can be rubbed along with the clitoris to produce enhanced sensation. However, the clitoris contains the highest concentration of nerve endings. There are no nerve endings in the vaginal canal itself. Pressure applied to some areas on the walls of the canal goes through the walls to stimulate nerves in tissues that surround the vagina. This pressure can be quite pleasurable depending on where and how the vaginal wall is stimulated, but unless a woman is regularly and easily experiencing clitoral orgasms, it would be unrealistic to expect her to experience orgasm by stimulation of spots on the vaginal wall.

This focus on the so-called *G-spot* may lead you to ignore the rest of your sensual potential and refrain from pleasurable research and experimentation into your own and your lover's sensual responses.

Dr. Leah M. Schwartz

95

Why should you improve your sex life?

Why should you aspire to do *anything* better? Sex is a wonderful gift worth investing in.

No one wants to believe that their last orgasm is the best they'll ever have.

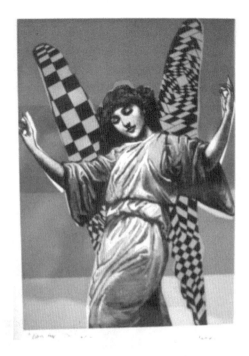

Who Taught You *That?*

96

Should I take it personally if my boyfriend masturbates?

Not at all. Sometimes a man masturbates to feel relaxed. If he believes that it's okay to masturbate, then he can do as he wishes.

If he enjoys orgasms, and wants to have more than he has with you, then you should let him unless it causes problems in your relationship.

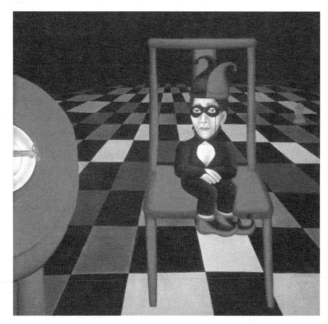

Dr. Leah M. Schwartz

97

How do I get the woman in my life to give me more oral sex?

Because your lover is obviously willing to perform oral sex, better find out from her what it is that she likes and doesn't like about doing it. Penetrating her mouth often triggers the gag reflex. You can prevent this by suggesting she wrap one or both lubricated hands (depending on length) around the shaft of your penis, thus giving her control of the amount of insertion and giving you full contact along the length of your penis.

She might also be more willing to do it if she doesn't feel the need to continue until you've ejaculated which may keep her working to the point of an aching jaw. She may also dislike the idea or the taste of your ejaculate in her mouth. In any one of these cases, you would have a hard time telling the difference in the dark between oral sex and a well-lubricated hand job.

You may be confusing the erotic with the sensual. It seems naughtier or more exciting to have a woman use her mouth because of social rules against one's mouth on people's genitals. Rather than trying to find a way to get her to do something she is uncomfortable with, find out from her what she is willing and unwilling to do and why. You cannot have nearly as much fun with someone who isn't having fun too.

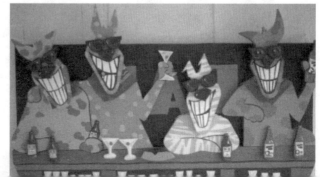

Who Taught You *That?*

98

How should I perform oral sex on my girlfriend?

The key to effective oral sex is a repetitious stroking motion of the clitoris with the tongue and gentle pressure with the lips. If you want to perform oral sex, what I recommend is that you ask for her permission. If you do it well the first time, *she will ask you again!*

Enjoying what you're doing is the very best thing you can do if her pleasure is your goal. Being fixated on ultimate results rather than immediate pleasure communicates to your lover the pressure of achievement and is consequently counterproductive.

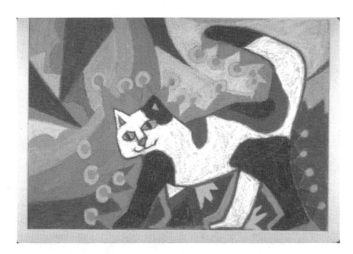

Dr. Leah M. Schwartz

99
What is the best way to introduce a new technique into your sexual relationship?

I would suggest that you ask your mate if he or she would like to try something new and fun in the sexual arena. Once you get a *yes*, let her or him know they are in charge, and any time they want to stop they can and you will honor their request.

The most important elements when trying something new sexually is to keep asking each step of the way and in each area. (1) Speed: start slow and experiment with different paces. (2) Direction: try different directions; up, down, sideway, around and around, left or right. Be willing to experiment and do what is most fun. (3) Pressure: start with light pressure and experiment with varying amounts. (4) Lubricant: once again small increments in all the areas I have mentioned.

For some of you, this suggestion may sound bizarre; however, great sex can be like a great meal. You can take *time outs* just like you can put your fork down in between wonderful bites of a meal. Remember the goal is fun and learning new sexual pleasures with and about each other.

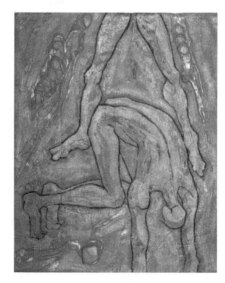

100

My partner feels that I need to satisfy him sexually, and I feel that he thinks that because he takes care of his responsibilities around the home, helps me with my children and financially provides, that my performing sex is like my payback to him. I know that sexually I am a bit conservative but I do not think that sex is a form of payment. I tell him that to stimulate me I have to have emotional and psychological well being. I am not like him. When I am having my period, I don't feel like getting intimate. He feels that he should not have to suffer for 4-5 days, so he will ask me to masturbate him or perform oral sex on him. This really upsets me because although I am not in the mood, he thinks that it is all about him. I feel like a whore at times. Help.

You are not a victim of bad luck. You have ended up with your standard kind of guy. He feels like he ought to get off at least every day and more often if possible. He thought that getting together with you would provide him with his idea of sensual gratification and in some ways, you must have led him to believe that this is what you would come up with. Otherwise, he wouldn't be doing all the the things he does to take care of you. Many women find themselves in exactly your spot. They know that guys are looking for regular sex and that if a woman can lead the guy to believe that he's going to get it from her she can arrange to have him stick around.

I know it sounds like a kind of barter or even prostitution, but women make themselves up, get their hair done, dress pretty and behave flirtatiously and sexily as a way to ensure that there will be a second date, a third date, and so on until the guy finally commits to being a reliable, dependable life partner. If the promise of sexual gratification is not included in the deal, the guy is unlikely to dedicate his life and productivity.

Dr. Leah M. Schwartz

When the courtship is over and the deal is done, many women find themselves shackled with the horrible obligation of sexual duty, as you do. The pleasure they had in the beginning of the relationship seems to have faded away. The sex they previously *liked* to do, they find they now *have* to do, and they don't want to do it.

Guys, on the other hand, understood that if they were going to score on a date, they would have to woo the woman. They would clean themselves up, dress nicely, take her out, treat her to fancy dinners, act nice, pay attention to her, compliment her, whisper sweet nothings and play the male part of seduction. Now that the deal is made, guys figure they've done what was necessary, so they abandon the role of the lover and adopt the role of the husband, figuring that if they come home sober with their paycheck they've got sex coming.

The way for you to get out of the hole you're in is to recognize that you don't want to be an asexual being—you want to be a woman. You can let out a little bit of spark for closeness and the guy will respond. Somehow you have to sit down with this guy and explain to him that he can't have any genuine fun unless you do as well.

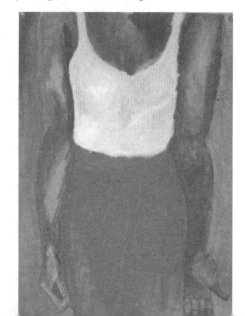

Make a contract that will give you both a goal to aim for. Orgasm is too low a goal for either of you. The only reasonable goal is that you both have fun using your bodies.

Who Taught You *That*?

101 *What is the ultimate sexual experience for a man?*

Providing a woman with the ultimate sexual experience.

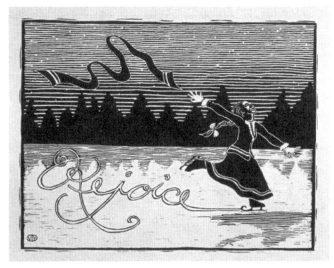

Dr. Leah M. Schwartz

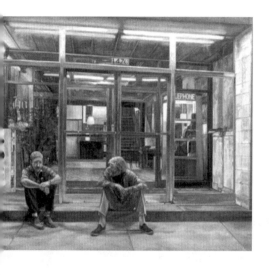

Dear Reader,

You've come to the end of my book of 101 important questions about sex, but I haven't nearly exhausted the hundreds of similar questions still remaining unanswered. In thousands of radio and television appearances, over a period of more than twenty years, you can imagine I have amassed quite a Q&A database.

If you've enjoyed this book, if it has helped you or brought you pleasure, you'll be pleased to know that I have every intention of writing another, with even more important questions about sex and sensuality. Look for it in your local bookstore, or drop me an e-mail (**drleah800@aol.com**) and I'll put you on a mailing list of announcements about upcoming products.

Thank you,

Dr. Leah M. Schwartz

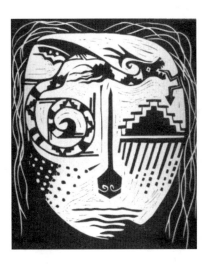

Where do I go if I need more help?

Many professionals earn their livelihood by producing dramatic results helping couples solve their relationship problems.

For a list of professionals, please write to:

The American Institute of Sexual Studies
Attention: Dr. Leah Schwartz
P.O. Box 2866
Houston, TX 77252-2866

Another possibility is to help yourself in the privacy of your home by using our series of sex education and self-help video tapes, DVDs and books, as described in the following pages.

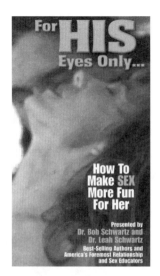

Just $39.95

Ask about special pricing when you buy two or more of any video or DVD.

Tape 1: For His Eyes Only...
How To Make Sex More Fun For Her

This video **(also available in DVD format)** is one of the best, most decent, tasteful, explicit, and effective adult romance and sex education videos ever produced for men. For the first time on video, several very different and attractive couples demonstrate "doing" the "Venus Butterfly" technique to a woman. This video brings The One Hour Orgasm to life for male viewers. It is filled with first-hand information that will improve any man's sexual effectiveness and his partner's sex life immediately.

• Improve your self confidence as a lover

• Increase the intensity and duration of her orgasms and cause her to have hundreds of orgasmic contractions

• Put the spark back, or prevent it from going away

• Bring back her sex drive

• Make every lovemaking session a pleasurable learning experience

• How even one inch of penetration can feel like twelve to her

• Solve the problem of not being in the mood at the same time

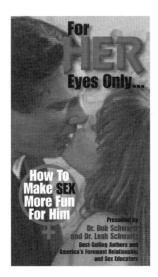

Just $39.95

Ask about special pricing when you buy two or more of any video or DVD.

Tape 2: For Her Eyes Only...
How To Make Sex More Fun For Him

This video **(also available in DVD format)** is one of the best sex education videos ever produced for women. For the first time on video, several very different and attractive couples demonstrate "doing" the "Venus Butterfly" technique to a man. This video brings The One Hour Orgasm to life for female viewers. It is filled with first-hand information that will improve any woman's sexual abilities.

- Improve your self-confidence as a lover
- Increase the intensity and duration of his orgasms
- Add 1 to 3 inches to his normal size
- Put the spark back, or prevent it from going away
- Bring back his sex drive
- Make every lovemaking session a pleasurable learning experience
- Learn "simulated" oral sex
- Solve the problem of not being in the mood at the same time
- Train his sexual nervous system to last longer

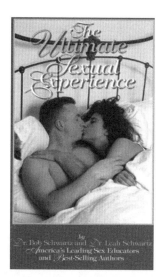

Just $39.95

Ask about special pricing when you buy two or more of any video or DVD.

Tape 3: The Ultimate Sexual Experience

This video (**also available in DVD format**) is the result of twenty years of incredible research by the nation's leading sex educators, Dr. Bob Schwartz and Dr. Leah Schwartz.

- Step-by-step to reaching sexual heights few even know exist!

- Is she really turned on?

- A "Touch of Ecstacy" that will leave her breathless!

- Footage never seen before of an incredible sexual phenomenon

- How even one inch of penetration can feel like twelve

- Learn to feel intensity you've never felt before

- Discover the common mistake most couples make

- The "Bread and Butter" stroke everyone is talking about

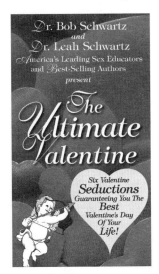

Just $39.95

Ask about special pricing when you buy two or more of any video or DVD.

Tape 4: The Ultimate Valentine

This video **(also available in DVD format)** features six romantic seductions to spice up any special occasion, including Valentine's Day, anniversaries, birthday, rainy weekends, or any time you just want to have some "special" fun! Featuring well-known models, including Griffen Drew from Playboy, and Penthouse magazine's Taylor St. Clair.

- Discover the "Velvet Touch" technique
- Learn how to inspire your Valentine to fulfill your wildest dreams!
- Get rid of your inhibitions, and use your Valentine's body to create the World's Sexiest Valentine!
- Discover your Valentine's hidden wild side
- Pamper your Valentine into fits of ecstacy!
- A must-have video!

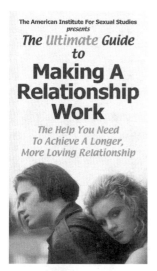

Tape 3: The Ultimate Guide To Making A Relationship Work

This unique and exciting video (**also available in DVD format**) is a must for everyone, whether contemplating a relationship or already in one. We take coaching for just about everything, but when it comes to one of the most important aspects of our lives, we think it's not necessary. This timely video will help you to:

- Discover how to build a lifetime relationship

- Repair damaged relationships

- Discover what your partner *really* wants

- Become more attractive to your partner

- Regain trust and avoid arguments

- Communicate better in, and out of, the bedroom

- Put the fun back into your relationship

- Even learn if your relationship is beyond repair

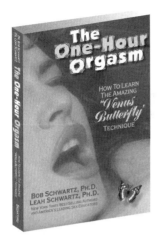

Just $12.95

Book 1: The One Hour Orgasm (Revised Third Edition)
How To Learn The Amazing "Venus Butterfly" Technique

Based on over 30 years of research and courses taught at More University and The Institute of Human Abilities in northern California, *The One-Hour Orgasm* is one of the best, most tasteful, explicit, and effective sex education books ever published. It demonstrates, with pictures and words, how you can master, to the delight of your sex partner, the famous "Venus Butterfly" technique, which promises an immediate improvement in your sex life.

The authors have discovered that if a couple were to "do" the "Venus Butterfly" to each other for as little as 3 minutes each week, it will do more to put the spark back in a relationship than an hour of therapy!

The One-Hour Orgasm is filled with fresh, easier to learn, new approaches and photos to aid the reader in learning the most effective lovemaking technique ever discovered.

Book 2: Diets Don't Work! (New, Entirely Revised Third Edition) Stop Dieting! Become "Naturally Thin" Live a Diet-Free Life

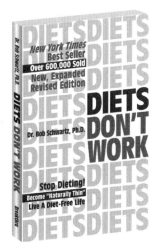

Just $12.95

If you are interested in losing weight and keeping it off for life, you'll want to order the *New York Times* best-selling book, *Diets Don't Work! Stop Dieting! Become "Naturally Thin" Live a Diet-Free Life* (Revised 3rd Edition) by Dr. Bob Schwartz.

Diets Don't Work! is recommended by universities and physicians all over the United States, Canada, and England.

• The real reasons you have not lost and kept it off;

• A method that is working for literally hundreds of millions of people in th world that keeps them thin without dieting;

• A new relationship with yourself, a new self-image based on you also being a "naturally thin" person;

• How to end your weight "problem" *once and for all.*

By reading this book, you will soon discover that you have taken the first step toward living the rest of your life without weight being an issue.

Ordering Information

For fastest service call our toll-free, 24-hour order line:
(800) 227-1152

All videos, DVDs and books are available for sale on the Internet. Visit **www.venusbutterfly.com** for all relationship self-help products, and **www.juststopdieting.com** for Diets Don't Work!

To order by mail, please write to:

Breakthru Publishing
P.O. Box 2866
Houston, TX 77252-2866

Just total your order and add a shipping charge of only $5.00 for as many items as you order (shipped to the same address).

Texas residents add 8.25% sales tax.

If you wish to receive your order by an expedited service, or to discuss discount pricing on quantity orders of our products for gifts or for resale, please call (800) 227-1152.

Sorry, no CODs.